CARDIOLOGY RESEARCH AND CLINICAL DEVELOPMENTS

DIETARY RISK FACTORS OF CARDIOVASCULAR DISEASES

Cardiology Research and Clinical Developments

Additional books in this series can be found on Nova's website
under the Series tab.

Additional e-books in this series can be found on Nova's website
under the e-book tab.

CARDIOLOGY RESEARCH AND CLINICAL DEVELOPMENTS

DIETARY RISK FACTORS OF CARDIOVASCULAR DISEASES

WENBIAO WU

NOVA BIOMEDICAL

New York

Additional color graphics may be available in the e-book version of this book.

Library of Congress Cataloging-in-Publication Data

ISBN: 978-1-63482-761-4

Library of Congress Control Number: 2015941526

Published by Nova Science Publishers, Inc. † New York

Contents

Preface

Although successful efforts have been greatly exerted to prevent and treat cardiovascular diseases (CVDs), it currently causes the most number of global deaths among all kinds of diseases. According to expert estimation in 2008, the global deaths caused by CVDs were 17.3 million, which accounted for 30% of all global deaths. Mathers and Loncar reported that the global deaths caused by CVDs could be up to 23.3 million by 2030. In addition to the global mortality of all CVDs, the World Health Organization (WHO) estimated that about 40% of adults aged 25 and over in the world suffer from hypertension. Hypertension greatly increases the risk of other kinds of CVDs that might be deadly. This means that CVDs result in many people's economical burdens and shortens their life span.

This book has comprehensively reviewed dietary risk factors for CVDs. There are several approved dietary risk factors for CVDs in our daily diets and foods. The dietary risk factors include toxicities caused by over-intake of cholesterol, energy, saturated fatty acids, saccharides (especially fructose), iron, sodium, alcohol, niacin, homocysteine, alkaloids (such as synephrines, caffeine, tyramine, dopamine, histamine, and cyanide), nucleic acids and trans-fatty acids. Other exstensive factors include the metabolites of choline-containing compounds or L-carnitine, and environmental contaminants such as mercury and cadmium; the deficiencies of folate and vitamins D, B_6, or B_{12}; the toxicity or deficiency of magnesium; and the consumption of sweetened soft drinks. Underweight—or even normal weight—individuals might not decrease the occurrence of cardiovascular diseases because the deficiency of some nutrients, and some alkaloids that are able to control weight could also damage the cardiovascular system.

It seems that the association of all these risk factors in blood with CVDs has been well established, though some controversial opinions on some risk factors exist. Also, their levels in blood are likely associated with their dietary intake. Therefore, it should be worth carrying out further studies on the correlation of these risk factors in foods with the occurrence of CVDs.

Most importantly, it seems that the data of dietary safety of these risk factors is based on a single factor. What would the cardiovascular system undergo if a person is used to foods that contain all cardiovascular risk factors for a long time? Is any unknown cardiovascular disease risk component present in our daily diets? It is worth performing extensive research to answer these questions. The disease risk factors on the cardiovascular system need to be studied well, even though the concentration of each in our daily food might be safe for consumption. For example, the test on a prepared diet containing all the risk factors for CVDs discussed in this book should have a prospective outcome and contribute a lot to the prevention of cardiovascular diseases in the future.

In addition, it has been reported that there are digoxin-like factors in some kinds of foods. Also, the association of the digoxin-like factors with CVDs has been indicated. For example, digoxin-like factors were found to cause bradycardia and hypotension, though they have been employed as medicines to enhance heart performance. Digoxin (1.2 ng/mL in blood and higher) may harm patients with heart failure. Its levels >2 ng/mL in blood are commonly toxic, but it may have toxicity at lower levels as well. Furthermore, digoxin especially harms patients who have significant sinus or atrioventricular block. A target range of 0.5-1.0 ng/dL in blood has been recommended.

It is believed that this book can be used as a reference for teachers, students, researchers, food or beverage manufacturers, food additive manufacturers, and those interested in healthy food.

Chapter 1

Introduction

Although successful efforts have been greatly exerted to prevent and treat cardiovascular diseases (CVDs), this kind of diseases currently causes the most number of global deaths among all kinds of diseases. According to expert estimation in 2008, the global deaths caused by CVDs were 17.3 million, which accounted for 30% of all global deaths [1]. Mathers and Loncar [2] reported that the global deaths caused by CVDs could be up to 23.3 million by 2030. In addition to the global mortality because of all CVDs, about 40% of adults aged 25 and over in the world suffered from hypertension in 2008 [3]. Hypertension greatly increases the risk of other kinds of CVDs that might be deadly.

The high prevalence of CVDs has currently become the serious problem not only in developed countries, but also in developing countries. CVDs are presently prevalent in both poor and rich people. CVDs could occur in people with regardless of ages though aged people may have greater risk of suffering from CVDs. They could also occur in people with regardless of sexes.

CVDs greatly result in economical burdens. The reason for this may be that it is quite difficult to cure a CVD relying on the current basis of available medical techniques developed. Once a CVD occurs, life time intake of drugs may usually be necessary for controlling it. Hypertension is a typical example. This kind of disease is very difficult to be cured so that the daily intake of blood pressure-lowering drugs may not be discontinued throughout lifetime.

CVDs are the chronic diseases that may finally determine on patient's life span. Generally, most old people (with ages ≥ 65 years) are likely to die of a chronic disease. At these ages, CVDs are the leading causes of deaths. For example, it is generally observed that blood vessels should stiffen with an increase in age. Until now, the present medical techniques available still seem to be incapable of replacing some damaged blood vessels (especially those in human brain) by healthy ones though the replacement of other organs (including a damaged heart) or tissues may be practicable. This should result from the complexity of the blood vessel system distributing in the human body.

Definition of CVDs

The cardiovascular system is responsible for transporting nutrients, hormones, gases (e.g. O_2 or CO_2), blood cells, wastes, etc. to and from cells throughout the body, which is also named circulatory system. Structurally, this system consists of heart, vessels and blood. Heart functions as a pump to push the circulation of blood held inside the vessels throughout the body, relying on the driving force resulting from the contraction and then relaxation of its muscles.

Heart and blood vessels may undergo structural damages, for example, the hypertrophy or fibrosis of heart, the deposition of undesirables on the surface of blood vessel endothelia, an increase in the stiffness or brokenness of blood vessels. The deposition of undesirables on the surface of blood vessel endothelia could cause serious conditions, such as atherosclerosis.

The structural damages of heart and blood vessels can result in their dysfunction. A CVD is usually defined as the dysfunction of heart and blood vessels. This kind of the dysfunction may result in hemorrhage and poor blood supply (e.g. hypertension, hypotension, or ischemia), depending upon the extent or variety of damages to the structure of heart or blood vessels. Hypertrophy or fibrosis in heart can decrease the efficiency of blood supply, such as an increase in hypotension or ischemia risk. An increase in the stiffness of blood vessels would elevate the risk of their brokenness and subsequently hemorrhage. The blockage by ruptured atherosclerotic plaques could result in ischemia. When hemorrhage or ischemia occurs in brain, it is defined as a stroke. When ischemia occurs in heart, it is defined as a heart attack.

Serious hemorrhage in brain or ischemia in both brain and heart could be deadly. These two illness conditions could be the outcome of chronic development of other CVDs.

Cardiac arrhythmias could be deadly sometimes though it is less common than heart attacks or strokes. This disease usually occurs when the electrical activity in the heart is abnormal. In this case, a too fast or too slow heartbeat that is regular or irregular may be observed. Palpitation or atrial fibrillation (one of the common tachyarrhythmias) belongs to this class of CVDs. (Each electrical impulse originated from the sino atrial node in the right atrium of the heart results in a heartbeat. An adult person at rest normally has about 70 (generally ranging from 60 to 100) times per minute heartbeats.)

Heart valve diseases (for example, aortic, mitral, tricuspid and pulmonary stenosis or insufficiency/regurgitation) are due to the abnormality of one or more of heart valves. A heart has four valves, i.e., mitral and aortic valves on its left as well as tricuspid and pulmonary valves on its right. This kind of disease is less common than heart attacks or strokes.

Heart muscle disease is a kind of cardiac dysfunction contributed by the progressive degeneration and weakness of skeletal muscles. Cardiomyopathy and muscular dystrophy belong to this class of CVDs. Although they do not commonly occur, the pathways of injuring and degenerating myocytes widely share in many varieties of illnesses.

Hypertension is a condition of too high blood pressure (systolic reading >140 mmHg or diastolic reading >90 mmHg) whereas hypotension refers to a too low blood pressure (a systolic reading <90 mmHg or a diastolic reading <60 mmHg). (An adult person at rest usually has a normal blood pressure ranging from 90 to 140 mmHg systolic reading and from 60 to 90 mmHg diastolic reading.) There are two types of hypertension, i.e. primary and secondary high blood pressure. The primary hypertension accounts for the 90–95% current morbidity of all hypertension cases [4]. The rest cases are secondary hypertension. Hypertension may not be acutely deadly and are usually controlled by drugs. However, it can increase the risk of other CVDs.

Biochemical Marks of CVDs

There are several biochemical marks of CVDs. The presence and accumulation of the biochemical marks may indicate the onset or risk of CVDs. Some CVDs may be the outcome of long term accumulation of the biochemical marks in the body or blood system.

The concentration of blood lipoprotein cholesterols is a critical indicating factor of some serious CVDs. High-, medium-, low- and very low-density lipoprotein cholesterols (HDLC, IDLC, LDLC and VLDLC, respectively) exist in blood. The lipoproteins are mainly packed with cholesterols. Until now, it can be certain that HDLC/LDLC (or TC) ratio is a critical indicator of atherosclerosis of blood vessels. That is to say that a lower HDLC/LDLC (or TC) ratio indicates a greater risk of developing atherosclerosis. Another important indicator is blood apolipoprotein (apo) A-I/apolipoprotein (apo) B (ApoA-I/ApoB) ratio. A lower blood ApoA-I/ApoB ratio indicates a higher possibility of developing atherosclerosis. The target and risk levels of HDLC/TC, HDLC/LDLC and ApoB/ApoA-I ratios for the primary and secondary prevention of atherosclerosis are shown in Table 1.

Increased levels of C-reactive protein (CRP), interleukin-6 (IL-6), tumor necrosis factor-α (TNF-α), and monocyte chemoattractant protein 1 (MCP 1), the activation of nuclear factor-κB (NF-κB), and the expression of cyclooxygenase 2 (Cox2) in blood may indicate the inflammation of the cardiovascular system. Furthermore, increased levels of soluble intercellular adhesion molecules (SICAMs), soluble vascular cell adhesion molecules (SVCAMs), and E-selectin in blood may indicate the endothelial dysfunction of blood vessels. Increased coagulant activity of factor VII may indicate the elevation of clot formation in the cardiovascular system. These would mean increases in the risk of developing CVDs.

Table 1. Target and risk levels of HDLC/TC, HDLC/LDLC and ApoB/ApoA-I ratios for the primary and secondary prevention of atherosclerosis [5-8]

Ratio	Secondary prevention				Primary prevention			
	Target level		Risk level		Target level		Risk level	
	Women	Men	Women	Men	Women	Men	Women	Men
HDLC/TC	>0.33	>0.29	<0.29	<0.25	>0.25	>0.22	<0.22	<0.2
HDLC/LDLC	>0.5	>0.4	<0.4	<0.33	>0.4	>0.33	<0.33	<0.29
ApoA-I/ApoB	>1.67	>1.43	<1.43	<1.25	>1.25	>1.11	<1.11	<1.0

Non-Dietary Causes of CVDs

The potential non-dietary factors of causing damages to heart or blood vessels might include viral or bacterial infections, physical damages, and genetic inheritance or mutation [9]. However, the morbidity of these non-dietary caused CVDs is normally very low except for hypertension. Here, the brief introduction of these CVDs is mainly for setting off the significance of dietary-related CVDs.

Rheumatic heart disease, mainly caused by rheumatic fever, only accounts for 1% of CVDs [10]. The rheumatic fever results from group A streptococcal bacteria infections. This kind of a CVD might occur in developing countries with widespread poverty. However, it can be treated or prevented by antibiotics (e.g. penicillin) or by the improvement of living conditions.

Normally, the physical damage of heart or blood vessels is very rare to occur. It may not be appropriate to regard the accidentally physical damage to heart or blood vessels as a CVD.

Many varieties of CVDs can occur due to genetic inheritance [11,12]. For example, the primary hypertension, the coronary artery disease (CAD) that is caused by blocking the arteries to provide blood to the heart, arrhythmogenic right ventricular or hypertrophic or dilated cardiomyopathies, and arrhythmias could be inherited.

The congenital heart disease (CHD), which is a heart condition with structural malformations observed at birth, may have several causing factors, including maternal malnutrition (such as shortage of folic acid) or infections (such as rubella) or use of drugs (such as warfarin) and alcohol, and a consanguineous marriage. Until now, the factors for causing such CHDs as abnormalities in heart chambers, abnormal valves and holes in the septum of the heart still remain unknown.

The primary hypertension could be caused by complicated interactions of environmental contributors, genes, and other factors, whose causes have not been exactly identified yet. Secondary hypertension could result from many other postnatal factors though it could also be associated with such diseases as Cushing's syndrome, pheochromocytoma, hypothyroidism, hyperthyroidism, acromegaly, hyperaldosteronism, hyperparathyroidism and renal disease [13], whose causes have been identified.

The Significance of Dietary Risk Factors of CVDs

Everyone needs appropriate amounts of energy and other essential nutrients including essential amino acids, fatty acids, vitamins and minerals for life existence every day. These nutrients cannot be synthesized by the human body and have to be provided by eating foods. The foods are digested in the digestive system (mainly stomach and intestine) and absorbable nutritional molecules are subsequently released. The absorbable nutrients should be absorbed into blood vessels through the mucosa mainly in the duodenum and the first part of jejunum except for vitamin B_{12} that is not absorbed before reaching the ileum. Only a tiny bit of nutrients may be absorbed in the stomach and the large intestine. Water soluble nutrients, e.g. amino acids, single sugars, water soluble vitamins or minerals should directly enter blood capillaries and then potal vein. Short-chain or some medium-chain free fatty acids and some monoacylglycerols enter the blood vessels and then via portal vein to the liver. Some free fatty acids (especially those with a long carbon chain), monoacylglycerols and other fatty compounds that are packed as chylomicrons enter the lymph system and then the blood circulation system (blood vessels and heart). Therefore, whether the long term contact of the nutrients with the endothelia of blood vessels or heart tissues is associated with CVDs or not should be well understood.

The growth of the cardiovascular system needs essential nutrients. The regeneration of damaged cardiovascular system or organs or tissues also needs essential nutrients. Therefore, it is also worth investigating whether the deficiency of essential nutrients is associated with CVDs or not.

People usually eat mixed foods. Even, every single food, such as potato, rice, bread, leafy vegetable, orange, has a very complex composition. Therefore, conventional foods contain not only essential nutrients, but also large amounts of non-nutritional components. Some of these non-nutritional components may be endogenous. Some others may be the contaminants from soils, atmosphere and irrigating water (including rainfall) in the growing area. Some of these non-nutritional components should also be absorbed into the circulation system (or called cardiovascular system). Once they enter the circulation system, they should contact with the endothelia of blood vessels or heart tissues. This means that it is very important to find out whether these non-nutritional components are associated with CVDs or not.

Majority of common CVDs may be associated with dietary factors. This means that dietary factors (including toxins and improper intake of certain nutrients) are critical for the prevention or even the treatment of a CVD. Even, the congenital heart disease may be prevented by optimizing women's diet before and throughout pregnancy [10]. Literature search shows that dietary risk factors for CVDs, including the overconsumption of cholesterols, energy, saturated fatty acids, saccharides (especially fructose), iron, sodium, alcohol, niacin, homocysteine, alkaloids (for example, synephrines, caffeine, tyramine, dopamine, histamine, and cyanide), nucleic acids, trans-fatty acids, and metabolites of choline-containing compounds (including phosphatidylcholine and L-carnitine) and such environmental contaminants as mercury or cadmium, and also the deficiencies of folate, vitamins D, B_6, or B_{12} as well as the improper consumption of magnesium and soda drink, have been identified. Since the low intake of some nutrients and alkaloids that are able to prevent the over-weight of the body could also damage the cardiovascular system, underweight or normal weight might not decrease the occurrence of CVDs. Therefore, the aim of this book was to comprehensively discuss these dietary risk factors for CVDs.

References

[1] WHO, Cardiovascular diseases fact sheet no.317. Geneva: World Health Organization; 2013. http://www.who.int/mediacentre/factsheets/fs317/en/. Accessed March 11, 2014

[2] Mathers, C.D., Loncar, D., (2006). Projections of global mortality and burden of disease from 2002 to 2030. *PLoS Med.* 3(11), e442.

[3] WHO, Global Health Observatory (GHO), Raised blood pressure. Geneva: World Health Organization; 2012. Available at: http://www.who.int/gho/ncd/risk_factors /blood_pressure_prevalence_ text/en/index.html. Accessed 6 December 2012

[4] Carretero, O.A., Oparil, S., (2000). Essential hypertension. Part I: definition and etiology. *Circulation* 101(3), 329–35.

[5] Millán, J., Pintó, X., Muñoz, A., Zúñiga, M., Rubiés-Prat, J., Pallardo, L.P., Masana, L., Mangas, A., Hernández-Mijares, A., González-Santos, P., Ascaso, J.F., Pedro-Botet, J., (2009). *Vasc. Health Risk Manag.* 5, 757–765.

[6] Holme, I., Aastveit, A.H., Junger, I., Walldius, G., (2008). Relationships between lipoprotein components and risk of myocardial infarction: age, gender and short versus longer follow-up periods in the Apolipoprotein Mortality Risk study (AMORIS). *J. Intern. Med.* 264, 30–38.

[7] Genest, J., Frohlich, J., Fodor, G., McPherson, R., (2003). the Working Group on Hypercholesterolemia and Other Dyslipidemias. Recommendations for the management of dyslipidemia and the prevention of cardiovascular disease: 2003 update. *CMAJ.* 169, 921–924.

[8] Gotto, A.M., Assmann, G., Carmena, R., Davignon, J., Fernandez-Cruz, , Fruchart, J.C., The ILIB lipid hand-book for clinical practice: blood lipids and coronary heart disease. 2nd ed. New York, NY: International Lipid Information Bureau; 2000; pp. 52, 53, 201.

[9] Wu, W., Sun, R., (2012). Toxicological studies of plant proteins: A review. *J. App. Toxicol.* 32(6), 377-464.

[10] Mendis, S., Puska, P., Norrving, B., Global atlas on cardiovascular disease: Prevention and control. Geneva: World Health Organization; 2011. ISBN 978 92 4 156437 3.

[11] Cirino, A.L., Ho, C.Y., (2013). Genetic Testing for Inherited Heart Disease. *Circulation* 128, e4-e8.

[12] Cambien, F., Tiret, L., (2007). Genetics of Cardiovascular Diseases: From Single Mutations to the Whole Genome. *Circulation* 116, 1714-1724.

[13] O'Brien, E., Beevers, D.G, Lip, G.Y.H., *ABC of hypertension.* London: BMJ Books; 2007. ISBN 1-4051-3061-X.

Chapter 2

Cholesterol

Cholesterol is a waxy steroid, which is quite different from a fat. The chemical name of cholesterol is 10,13-dimethyl-17-(6-methylheptan-2-yl)-2,3,4,7,8,9,11,12,14,15,16,17-dodecahydro-1H-cyclopenta[a]phe-nanthren-3-ol. Its molecular weight is 386.65 g/mol. Its solubility in water is negligible (only about 0.096 mg/L at 30°C). It is soluble in ethanol, methanol, acetone, benzene, isopropyl myristate, hexane, ether, and chloroform. The molecular structure diagram of the cholesterol is shown in Figure 1.

The cholesterol was first found in gallstones in 1769 by François Poulletier de la Salle and Eugène Chevreul who first named this compound "cholesterine" in 1815 [1]. The word “cholesterol” was derived from the *chole*-(bile) consecutively followed by the *stereos* (solid) and *ol* (alcohol).

The cholesterol exists not only in human gallstones, but also in the liver, brain, and blood. It is essential for constructing mammalian cell membranes and is necessary for establishing appropriate membrane fluidity or permeability. It is also a precursor for biosynthesizing bile acids, vitamin D and steroid hormones [2].

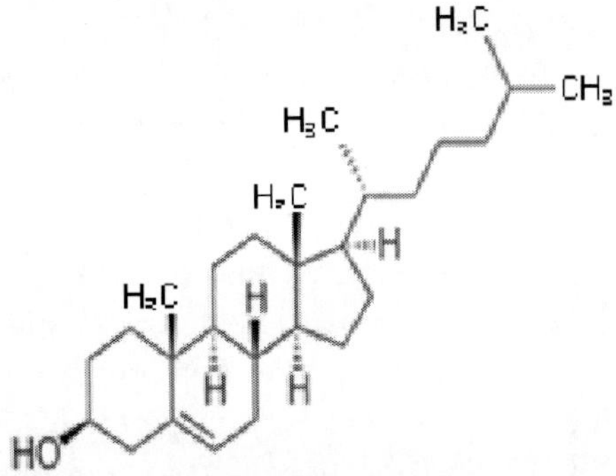

Figure 1. Cholesterol.

The cholesterol can be created inside the human body. Animal studies involving rats or puppies also indicated that diets free of cholesterols didn’t result in any symptom of deficiency. There is a mechanism of biochemical feedback in liver cells in order to avoid the synthesis of cholesterols over the amount that is required. The reason for this is that the biosynthesis of cholesterols is very energy-intensive. This feedback mechanism needs a key component, i.e. the enzyme, called 3-hydroxy-3-methylglutaryl coenzyme A (HMG-CoA) reductase. In case of lacking cholesterols, the irreversible jumpstarting of producing it needs a chemical conversion that requires the catalysis of HMG-CoA reductase. However, the activity of HMG-CoA reductase should be shut down by a key enzyme that is triggered by adequate amounts of cholesterols in the liver. This biochemical process eventually stops the biosynthesis of cholesterols. Therefore, the cholesterol in foods or diets would reduce its biosynthesis in the body if it is absorbed. The danger of eating cholesterol-rich foods would be that the over-absorption of cholesterols than that they are needed by the body cannot be stopped by the homeostatic mechanism. It is very difficult to control the amount of cholesterols eaten and absorbed being just equal to that it is needed by the body.

Absorption of Cholesterol

In the gut lumen, there are cholesterols, derived from diets and bile (ca. 1 g/day). These cholesterols are usually not absorbed completely in humans. The average absorption rate of the cholesterols in the gut lumen is only about 50% whereas the rest is discarded with the faeces. However, the absorption rates of the cholesterols are widely different between individuals, and they in percentages range from 15 to 75% [3]. The absorption of cholesterols is also regulated by genetic and metabolic factors so that the response to its variations in diets or foods is very different in individuals.

After the cholesterols are released by digestion, the absorption of the cholesterols is relied on forming micelles with the bile salts like the digestion. This is due to that the solubility of the cholesterols in the aqueous environment of the gut is very poor. If the cholesterols in the foods are esterified, they cannot form micelles with the bile salts. Once the cholesterols are released by the esterase hydrolyzation, they can participate into bile acid micelles. Usually, the esterified cholesterols account for 10–15% of total cholesterols in the food. A formed micelle is a mixture of free cholesterols, bile acids, phospholipids, lysophospholipids, fatty acids, monoacylglycerides, and triglycerides. The hydrophilic groups of these lipid complexes positioned outside the micelle facilitate its penetration through the unstirred aqueous layer. This aqueous layer at the enterocyte-intestinal lumen interface is a barrier for diffusion. Further work is needed to understand the exact mechanism of the unesterified cholesterol-containing micelles subsequently crossing the brush-border membrane of mucosa and being taken up by the mucosal cells. It was believed that the absorption of the cholesterols is a diffusion process that is passive, energy-independent, and simple [4]. For the absorption of the cholesterols, it was reported that there are three key proteins involved, i.e., Niemann Pick C1 like 1 (NPC1L1) as a cholesterol-uptaking transporter [5], and ATP-binding cassette (ABC) proteins ABCG5 and ABCG8 as cholesterol efflux transporters [6].

The absorption of the cholesterols is greatly inhibited by the presence of some other compounds in the foods. The absorption rate of dietary cholesterols may be reduced by the presence of such food components as excessive phospholipids though biliary phospholipids are very important for cholesterols being effectively solved in the bile and phytosterols [7]. For example, studies on young healthy rats indicated that phosphatidylcholines reduced the absorption of cholesterols [8]. Animal studies indicated that the absorption of dietary cholesterols was reduced 50% and 40% by phytosphingosines and sphingolipids having a structure similar to that of phytosphingosines, respectively [9]. Vegetable oils and their further processed products are the richest phytosterol sources that naturally exist. Phytosterols are also rich in nuts. Stigmasterol, campesterol and β-sitosterol are the phytosterols the most commonly found in the human foods, which account for ca. 3%, 30%, and 65% of dietary supplies, respectively [10].

It should also be noted that the cholesterol-lowering effect of phospholipids may be counteracted by such factors as elder age with type 2 diabetes [11].

Transporting Forms of Cholesterol

In the body, cholesterols are packaged as high-density lipoproteins (HDLC), low-, intermediate- or very low-density lipoprotein-cholesterol (LDLC, IDLC and VLDLC, respectively) for transportation in the circulatory system. The particle size of these lipoproteins, from the smallest to the largest in order, is high density lipoprotein (HDL), low-density lipoprotein (LDL), intermediate-density lipoprotein (IDL), and very low-density lipoprotein (VLDL). The particle size of all the lipoproteins mentioned above is smaller than that of chylomicrons. The size of all these lipoprotein particles is smaller than that of human cells. These lipoproteins consist of multiple proteins combined with fatty substances and subsequently formed complex particles that transport all lipids (fatty molecules) around the body in the aqueous environment outside cells.

A HDL particle typically consists of 80-100 proteins (with 1, 2 or 3 ApoA as organizers). More ApoAs are picked up as the particle enlarges as well as picking up more fat molecules. Therefore, none to hundreds fat molecules would be transported by a HDL particle. The proportion of proteins to lipids is the highest in a HDL particle so that it is the densest among all kinds of lipoproteins. ApoA-I (the major one) and ApoA-II are the most abundant apolipoproteins in a HDL particle. APOA1 gene in humans encodes ApoA-I [12,13]. This protein has 28.1 kDa molecular weight [14]. It has recently been suggested that an endogenously expressed antisense RNA regulates APOA1 mRNA [15]. There is biochemically an extra cysteine bridge in an ApoA-I molecule. This results in its existence as a heterodimer or as a homodimer with ApoA-II that has 17.4 kDa molecular weight [14]. The ApoA-I is able to enhance lipid (including cholesterol) efflux from tissues to the liver for being excreted. This protein is a cofactor for lecithin cholesterolacyltransferase (LCAT) which also needs the ApoA-I as a cofactor for forming most blood cholesteryl esters. The function of HDL particles is responsible for the removal of lipid molecules from cells that need to export these lipids. The lipids transported include triglycerides, phospholipids and cholesterols. The amounts of each of these lipids in a HDL particle vary considerably. The ApoA-I was also reported to be a factor of stabilizing prostacyclin (PGI2) and therefore might possess an anti-clotting effect [16].

A LDL particle typically consists of 80-100 proteins (with a single ApoB as an organizer). It can carry ca. 3,000-6,000 lipid molecules. The most abundant protein of the ApoB group is ApoB-100 that is composed of 4563 amino acids and has 514 kDa molecular weight though ApoB48 was also found in the plasma [17]. Therefore, a LDL particle normally consists of a single ApoB-100 molecule as well as additional 80 to 100 of other proteins. Hundreds to thousands (an average of ca. 1500) non-esterified and esterified cholesterol molecules, polyunsaturated fatty acids (i.e. linoleates), triglycerides and other lipids together form the highly hydrophobic core in a LDL particle. A shell of the single copy of Apo B-100, unesterified cholesterols and phospholipids surrounds this hydrophobic core. The lipids transported by a LDL particle include triglycerides, phospholipids and cholesterols. The amounts of each of these lipids in a LDL particle vary considerably. The diameter of a LDL particle is ca. 0.00000087 in. (22 nm) and its mass is ca. 3 million daltons. However, the size and mass of a LDL particle may vary since different LDL particles contain variable number of different fatty acid molecules [18]. The movement of lipids around the body within the aqueous environment outside cells is enabled by each native LDL particle that carries all fatty acids being surrounded and packed or emulsified.

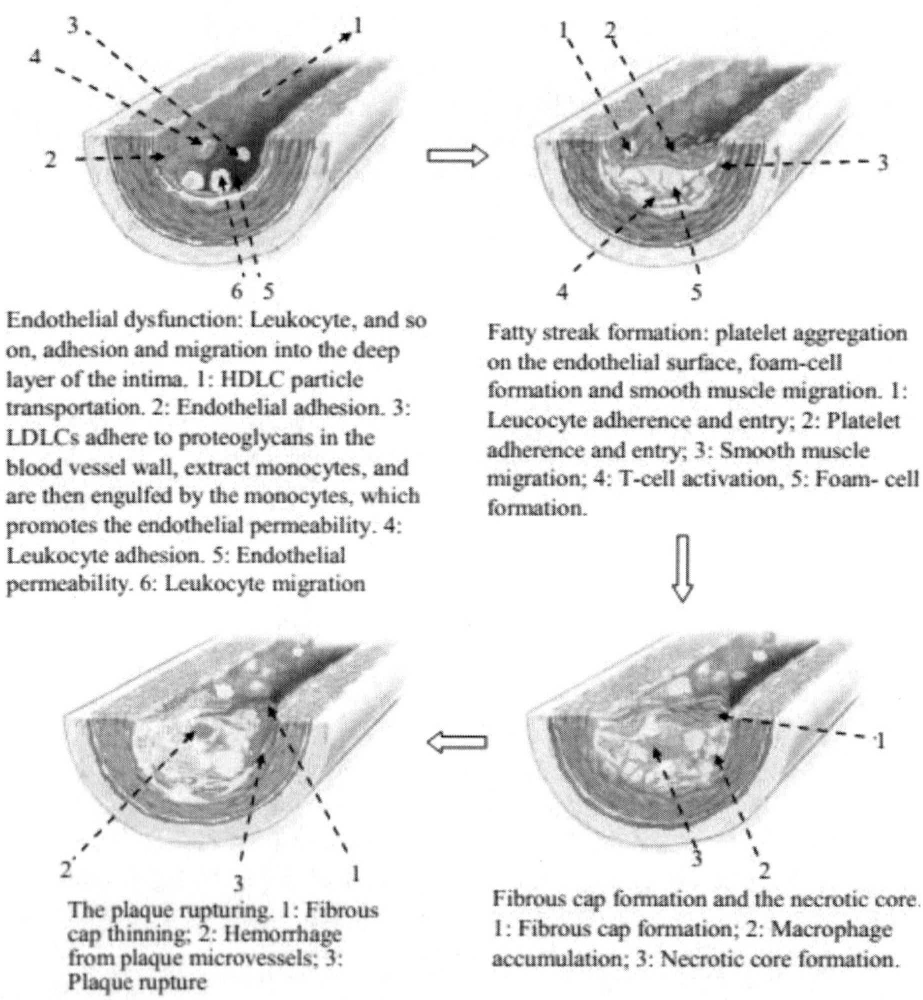

Figure 2. Mechanism of blood clot formation initiated by LDLCs [26].

An IDL particle is the degrading product of a VLDL. In addition to a single copy of ApoB-100A, an IDL particle possesses multiple copies of the receptor ligand apolipoprotein E (ApoE). The diameter of an IDL particle is ca. 25 to 35 nm. An IDL particle primarily consists of a range of cholesterols and triacylglycerols esters and can be further converted to a

LDL particle by triglyceride hydrolysis. The multiple copies of ApoE in an IDL particle have very high affinity of binding to the LDL receptor. When only the ApoB-100 stays in and the ApoE is removed from the IDL particle, it is transferred to a LDL particle whose affinity for the LDL receptor is much decreased [19]. ApOE contains 299 amino acids [20]. It is polymorphic [21,22], with three major alleles found, i.e. ApoE2 (cys112, cys158), ApoE3 (cys112, arg158), and ApoE4 (arg112, arg158) [23]. The function of ApoE is for transporting cholesterols, fat-soluble vitamins, and lipoproteins consecutively into the lymph and then blood systems. This protein is created mainly in the liver, but also exists in such other tissues as the spleen, kidneys and brain.

A VLDL particle initially produced in the liver consists of triglycerides, cholestryl esters, cholesterols, ApoB-100, apolipoprotein C1 (ApoC1, consisting of 57 amino acids) that is encoded by ApoC1 gene in humans [24], and ApoE. Once a nascent VLDL particle enters the blood circulatory system, it starts to have apolipoprotein C-II (ApoC-II) and additional ApoE donated from a HDL joining in the particle. Subsequently, the nascent VLDL is converted to a mature VLDL. The diameter of the VLDL particle is 30-80 nm. When a VLDL in blood circulates, it meets up a protein lipoprotein lipase (LPL) in the capillary beds of the tissues (skeletal muscle, adipose, or cardiac). Triglycerides in the VLDL particle will be removed by the LPL for storing or producing energy. Then, the VLDL particle comes back in contact with a HDL particle that picks up back the ApoC-II from the VLDL particle whereas ApoE remains. Cholesteryl esters are also transferred to the VLDL by the HDL in exchange for triglycerides as well as phospholipids through a cholesterylester transfer protein (CETP). As the LPL and CETP enzymes remove more and more triglycerides from the VLDL particle, the VLDL is converted to an IDL because of the changes in molecular composition [25].

Dietary Cholesterol and Risk of CVDs

LDLCs or VLDLCs trigger the deposition of the plaque in blood vessels, which are believed to be bad cholesterols. The mechanism of LDLCs or VLDLCs involved in atherosclerosis is summarized in Figure 2. Presently, it is generally believed that an excessive amount of LDLCs circulating in the blood is responsible for starting up the development of atherosclerosis. The excessive LDLCs in the blood could be induced by diets though a genetic tendency could also be a factor. The excess of LDLCs would promote some of them to transport into the space between the cells that constitute the inner walls of arteries. This conclusion was further extended by Frank and Fogelman [27] who indicated the rapid transportation of LDL particles across an intact endothelium by using ultra-structural techniques and the LDL particles are caught in the trap of the three-dimensional cage being composed of fibrils as well as fibers released by the cells of the artery wall [28]. These results are consistent with the fact that the ApoB (the major apolipoprotein in a LDL particle) concentration is higher in the artery wall than in the blood [29-31]. It was also reported that lipoproteins lodged in the wall of artery were more important than their rate transported into the wall of artery for any given concentration of lipoproteins in the blood [32, 33]. The LDLC particles trapped cannot be easily destructed and therefore continue lodging in between these cells. The oxidative products released by the cells of the artery wall via several pathways initiate the oxidation of lipids in the LDL particle trapped in the subendothelial space [34-37].

These processes would result in a local irritation. To remove the irritating LDL particles, the macrophages (the cells of the immune system responsible for eating garbages) are allured into the lodged LDLCs in the subendothelial space of the artery wall for ingesting them. Some macrophages expire eventually and release their cholesterols ingested into the wall of the artery. The cholesterols released by the dead macrophages conjugate with the macrophages that are engorged by intact cholesterols and result in the fatty streaks in the arteries. A tough cellular patch is often formed when a wound allures its surrounding fibrous muscle cells into it. A fatty streak that is laden by cholesterols also allures these muscle cells into it so that a fibrous plaque forms. The plaques formed result in thickening, narrowing, and even stiffening arteries. The narrowed artery is not able to supply the heart with sufficient amount of blood that is laden by oxygen and therefore causes angina (chest pain). As time goes on, some serious plaques are likely to fragment and result in clots in the blood. The clots can block the flow of blood into the heart or brain, which can cause angina (or a heart attack) or stroke, respectively.

HDLCs remove LDLCs or VLDLCs from arterial walls. HDLCs are therefore believed to be good cholesterols. This conclusion mainly result from the fact that HDLs carry cholesterols out of the regions that are injured by cholesterols in the arteries and transport them into the liver that safely stores or destroys them. HDLs are also able to protect the artery from the lodgement of cholesterols and the formation of plagues that are promoted by the influx of muscle cells and macrophages. Therefore, the HDLCs are beneficial to the prevention of CVDs.

An increase in the HDLC/LDLC or (LDLC+VLDLC) ratio in blood is negatively correlated with the occurrence or even mortality of CVDs (also see Table 1 in *Chapter 1*). Therefore, a diet that elevates LDLCs or VLDLCs and decreases HDLCs potentially increases the risk of CVDs [38]. A meta-analysis of studies on subjects ranged from 18 to 75 years old indicated that increased dietary cholesterols (100 mg/day) decreased the HDLC/LDLC or (LDLC+VLDLC) ratio (0.02 units). It was also reported that the modest elevation of LDLC concentration in the blood was achieved by a net increase in cholesterols supplied to the liver [39]. A report on the experimental results obtained by feeding rabbits for 12 weeks, which was published in 2013 by Hur et al. [40], concluded that dietary cholesterols (CHOs) and cholesterol oxides added did not affect the HDLC levels in the serum of rabbits, but induced atherosclerotic lesions. However, the HDLC/LDLC ratio should be a better index of predicting the risk of CVDs. Therefore, it should be noted that the HDLC/LDLC ratio is negatively correlated with the amount of dietary cholesterols plus cholesterol oxides added (see Table 2). This result indicates that an increase in the intake of cholesterols in diets may significantly decrease the HDLC/LDLC ratio that well predicts the risk of developing CVDs.

The research to date is controversial on the effect of reducing cholesterol intake on blood cholesterol level or the occurrence of CVDs. The maximum daily cholesterol intake <300 mg for healthy individuals has been recommended [41], whereas the EFSA Panel on Dietetic Products, Nutrition, and Allergies has not proposed a reference value of daily cholesterol intake [42]. Furthermore, a contradictory conclusion of an investigation on children aged 8-12 years (who ate 2 eggs/day) also appeared in the literature [43].

The controversial results mentioned above might be explained by the coexistence of other factors. The coexistence of dietary cholesterols and fats or oils, which is the case for most animal foods, may be a factor in the subsequent induction of CVDs. Preconditioning the same cholesterol level in all diets, the lymph cholesterol level (20-30% in LDLC and VLDLC particles) in rats fed coconut oil was the highest, while that in rats fed corn oil was in the middle and that in rats fed sesame oil was the lowest [44]. Also, the intake of vitamin C tends to increase HDLCs in the blood.

In a rare case, hypocholesterolemia (<100 mg/dL in blood serum) may not mean a healthy condition. However, this poor condition is usually associated with serious diseases rather than the under-intake of dietary cholesterols [45-48].

Table 2. Effect of dietary cholesterols (CHOs) and cholesterol oxides (COPs) on the HDLC/LDLC ratio in the serum of rabbits fed for 12 weeks

Dietary CHOs + COPs (g/kg diet)	HDLC/LDLC ratio
0 g	2.72
0.51 g CHOs + 0.49 COPs	0.29
0.81 g CHOs + 0.19 COPs	0.28
0.91 g CHOs + 0.09 COPs	0.12
1.0 g CHOs	0.12
1.21 g CHOs + 0.79 COPs	0.11
1.61 g CHOs + 0.39 COPs	0.052
2 g CHOs	0.050

Table 3. The list of top foods having the highest cholesterol content (mg/100 g edible food portion) **[49]**

Food sources	Cholesterol content
Beef	262.00 (variety meats and by-products, pancreas, cooked, braised) - 3100.00 (variety meats and by-products, brain, cooked, simmered)
Veal	263.00 (variety meats and by-products, lungs, cooked, braised) - 3100.00 (variety meats and by-products, brain, cooked, braised)
Pork	277.00 (fresh, variety meats and by-products, chitterlings, cooked, simmered) - 2552.00 (fresh, variety meats and by-products, brain, cooked, braised)
Lamb	284.00 (variety meats and by-products, lungs, cooked, braised) - 2504.00 (variety meats and by-products, brain, cooked, pan-fried)
Egg	352.00 (whole, cooked, scrambled) - 2335.00 (yolk, dried)
Fish oil	485.00 (salmon) - 766.00 (herring)
Fish,	266.00 (whitefish, dried (Alaska Native)) - 588.00 (caviar, black and red, granular)
Chicken	262.00 (broilers or fryers, giblets, raw) - 564.00 (liver, all classes, cooked, pan-fried)
Duck,	515.00 (domesticated, liver, raw)
Goose	515.00 (liver, raw)
Turkey	282.00 (all classes, giblets, raw) - 388.00 (liver, all classes, cooked, simmered)
Moose	389.00 (liver, braised (Alaska Native))

Cholesterol-Rich Foods

Cholesterols are mainly present in such animal food resources as cheese, egg yolk, beef, pork, poultry, fish and shrimp. The list of top foods having the highest cholesterol content is shown in Table 3. The data shown in the table are extracted from USDA National Nutrient

Database for Standard Reference Release 27 [49]. Their quantities in human breast milk are also significant.

Cholesterols are normally absent in plant food resources. The intake of some plant foods may be a good way to reduce blood cholesterols.

References

[1] Olson, R.E., (1998). Discovery of the lipoproteins, their role in fat transport and their significance as risk factors. *J. Nutr.* 128(2 Suppl), 439S-443S.

[2] Hanukoglu, I., (1992). Steroidogenic enzymes: structure, function, and role in regulation of steroid hormone biosynthesis. *J. Steroid. Biochem. Mol. Biol.* 43(8), 779-804.

[3] Grundy, S.M., (1983). Absorption and metabolism of dietary cholesterol. *Annu. Rev. Nutr.* 3, 71-96.

[4] Wilson, M.D., Rudel, L.L., (1994). Review of cholesterol absorption with emphasison dietary and biliary cholesterol. *J. Lipid Res.* 35, 943-955.

[5] Davis, H.R., Altmann, S.W., (2009). Niemann-PickC1 Like 1 (NPC1L1) an intestinal sterol transporter. *Biochim. Biophys. Acta* 1791, 679-683.

[6] Sabeva, N.S., Liu, J., Graf, G.A., (2009). The ABCG5 ABCG8 sterol transporter and phytosterols: implications for cardiometabolic disease. *Curr. Opin. Endocrinol. Diabetes Obes.* 16, 172-177.

[7] Racette, S.B., Lin, X., Lefevre, M., Spearie, C.A., Most, M.M., Ma, L., Ostlund, R.E., (2010). Dose effects of dietary phytosterols on cholesterol metabolism: a controlled feeding study. *Am. J. Clin. Nutr.* 91, 32–8.

[8] Jiang, Y., Noh, S.K., Koo, S.I., (2001). Egg phosphatidylcholine decreases the lymphatic absorption of cholesterol in rats. *J. Nutr.* 131, 2358 –2363.

[9] Duivenvoorden, I., Voshol, P.J., Rensen, P.C., van Duyvenvoorde, W., Romijn, J.A., Emeis, J.J., Havekes, L.M., Nieuwenhuizen, W.F., (2006). Dietary sphingolipids lower plasma cholesterol and triacylglycerol and prevent liver steatosis in APOE*3 Leiden mice. *Am. J. Clin. Nutr.* 84, 312-321.

[10] Weihrauch, J.L., Gardner, J.M., (1978). Sterol content of foods of plant origin. *J. Am. Diet. Assoc.* 73(1), 39–47.

[11] Houston, D.K., Ding, J., Lee, J.S., Garcia, M., Kanaya, A.M., Tylavsky, F.A., Newman, A.B., Visser, M., Kritchevsky, S.B., (2011). Dietary fat and cholesterol and risk of cardiovascular disease in elder adults: The health ABC study. *Nutr. Metab. Cardiovasc. Dis.* 21(6), 430–437.

[12] Breslow, J., Ross, D., McPherson, J., Williams, H., Kurnit, D., Nussbaum, A.L., Karathanasis, S.K., Zannis, V.I., (1982). Isolation and characterization of cDNA clones for human apolipoprotein A-I. *Proc. Natl. Acad. Sci. U.S.A.* 79(22), 6861–5.

[13] Arinami, T., Hirano, T., Kobayashi, K., Yamanouchi, Y., Hamaguchi, H., (1990). Assignment of the apolipoprotein A-I gene to 11q23 based on RFLP in a case with a partial deletion of chromosome 11, del(11)(q23.3----qter). *Hum. Genet.* 85(1), 39–40.

[14] Massey, J.B., Pownall, H.J., Macha, S., Morris, J., Tubb, M.R., Silva, R.A.G.D., (2009). Mass spectrometric determination of apolipoprotein molecular stoichiometry in reconstituted high density lipoprotein particles. *J. Lipid Res.* 50(6), 1229–1236.

[15] Halley. P., Kadakkuzha, B., Faghihi, M., Magistri, M., Zeier, Z., Khorkova, O., Coito, C., Hsiao, J., Lawrence, M., Claes Wahlestedt, C., (2014). Regulation of the Apolipoprotein Gene Cluster by a Long Noncoding RNA. *Cell Rep.* 6(1), 222–230.

[16] Yui. Y., Aoyama, T., Morishita, H., Takahashi, M., Takatsu, Y., Kawai, C., (1988). Serum prostacyclin stabilizing factor is identical to apolipoprotein A-I (apo A-I). A novel function of apo A-I. *J. Clin. Invest.* 82(3), 803–7.

[17] Chen, S.H., Yang, C.Y., Chen, P.F., Setzer, D., Tanimura, M., Li, W.H., Gotto, A.M., Chan, L., (1986). The complete cDNA and amino acid sequence of human apolipoprotein B-100. *J. Biol. Chem.* 261(28), 12918–12921.

[18] Segrest, J.P., Jones, M.K., De Loof, H., Dashti, N., (2001). Structure of apolipoprotein B-100 in low density lipoproteins. *J. Lipid Res.* 42(9), 1346–67.

[19] Brown, M.S., Goldstein, J.L., (1986). A receptor-mediated pathway for cholesterol homeostasis. *Science* 232, 34–47.

[20] Singh, P.P., Singh, M., Mastana, S.S., (2002). Genetic variation of apolipoproteins in North Indians. *Hum. Biol.* 74(5), 673–82.

[21] Singh, P.P., Singh, M., Mastana, S.S., (2006). APOE distribution in world populations with new data from India and the UK. *Ann. Hum. Biol.* 33(3), 279–308.

[22] Eisenberg, D.T., Kuzawa, C.W., Hayes, M.G., (2010). Worldwide allele frequencies of the human apoliprotein E (APOE) gene: climate, local adaptations and evolutionary history. *Am. J. Phys. Anthropol.* 143(1), 100–111.

[23] Ghebranious, N., Ivacic, L., Mallum, J., Dokken, C., (2005). Detection of ApoE E2, E3 and E4 alleles using MALDI-TOF mass spectrometry and the homogeneous mass-extend technology. *Nucleic Acids Res.* 33(17), e149.

[24] Tata, F., Henry, I., Markham, A.F., Wallis, S.C., Weil, D., Grzeschik, K.H., Junien, C., Williamson, R., Humphries, S.E., (1985). Isolation and characterisation of a cDNA clone for human apolipoprotein CI and assignment of the gene to chromosome 19. *Hum. Genet.* 69(4), 345–9.

[25] Shelness, G.S., Sellers, J.A., (2001). Very-low-density lipoprotein assembly and secretion. *Curr. Opin. Lipidol.* 12(2), 151–157.

[26] Ross, R., (1999). Mechanisms of disease: Atherosclerosis – an inflammatory disease. *N. Engl. J. Med.* 340, 115–126.

[27] Frank, J.S., Fogelman, A.M., (1989). Ultrastructure of the intima in WHHL and cholesterol-fed rabbit aortas prepared by ultra-rapid freezing and freeze-etching. *J. Lipid Res.* 30, 967-978.

[28] Nievelstein, P.F.E.M., Fogelman, A.M., Mottino, G., Frank, J.S., (1991). Lipid accumulation in rabbit aortic intima 2 hours after bolus infusion of low density lipoprotein: a deep-etch and immunolocalization study of rapidly frozen tissue. *Arterioscler. Thromb.* 11, 1795-1805.

[29] *Smith, E.B., (1974). The relationship between plasma and tissue lipids in human atherosclerosis. Adv. Lipid Res.* 12, 1-49.

[30] *Hoff, H.F., Heideman, C.L., Gaubatz, J.W., Gotto, A.M., Erickson, E.E., Jackson, R.L., (1977). Quantification of apolipoprotein B in grossly normal human aorta. Circ. Res.* 40, 56-64.

[31] *Hoff, H.F., Heideman, C.L., Gotto, A.M., Gaubatz, J.W., (1977). Apolipoprotein B retention in the grossly normal and atherosclerotic human aorta. Circ. Res.* 41, 684-*690.*

[32] *Schwenke, D.C., Carew, T.E., (1989). Initiation of atherosclerotic lesions in cholesterol-fed rabbits, I: focal increases in arterial LDL concentrations precede development of fatty streak lesions. Arterioscler.* 9, 895-*907.*

[33] *Schwenke, D.C., Carew, T.E., (1989). Initiation of atherosclerotic lesions in cholesterol-fed rabbits, II: selective retention of LDL vs selective increases in LDL permeability in susceptible sites of arteries. Arterioscler.* 9, 908-*918.*

[34] *Witztum, J.L., Steinberg, D., (1991). Role of oxidized low density lipoprotein in atherogenesis. J. Clin. Invest.* 88, 1785-*1792.*

[35] Parthasarathy, S., Modified Lipoproteins in the Pathogenesis of Atherosclerosis. Austin, Tex: RG Landes Co; 1994; pp.91-119.

[36] Parthasarathy, S., Mechanism(s) of cell-mediated oxidation of low density lipoprotein. In: Nohl H, Esterbauer H, Rice Evans C, eds. Free Radicals in the Environment, Medicine and Toxicology. London, England: Richelieu Press; 1994; pp.163-179.

[37] *Witztum, J.L., (1994). The oxidation hypothesis of atherosclerosis. Lancet.* 344, 793-*795.*

[38] Weggemans, R.M., Zock, P.L., Katan, M.B., (2001). Dietary cholesterol from eggs increases the ratio of total cholesterol to high-density lipoprotein cholesterol in humans: a meta-analysis. *Am. J. Clin. Nutr.* 73, 885–891.

[39] Spady, D.K., Woollett, L.A., Dietschy, J.M., (1993). Regulation of plasma LDL-cholesterol levels by dietary cholesterol and fatty acids. *Annu. Rev. Nutr.* 13, 355-81.

[40] Hur, S.J., Min, B., Nam, K.C., Lee, E.J., Ahn, D.U., (2013). Effect of Dietary Cholesterol and Cholesterol Oxides on Blood Cholesterol, Lipids, and the Development of Atherosclerosis in Rabbits. *Int. J. Mol. Sci.* 14, 12593-12606.

[41] USDA and USDHHS (U.S. Department of Agriculture and U.S. Department of Health and Human Services), Dietary guidelines for Americans, 2010, 7th Edition. Washington, D.C., U.S.: Government Printing Office; 2010.

[42] EFSA., (2010). Scientific opinion on dietary reference values for fats, including saturated fatty acids, polyunsaturated fatty acids, monounsaturated fatty acids, trans fatty acids, and cholesterol. *EFSA J.* 8(3), 1461.

[43] Ballesteros, M.N., Cabrera, R.M., Saucedo, M.S., Fernandez, M.L., (2004). Dietary cholesterol does not increase biomarkers for chronic disease in a pediatric population from northern Mexico. *Am. J. Clin. Nutr.* 79, 213–217.

[44] Satchithanandam, S., Reicks, M., Calvert, R.J., Cassidy, M.M., Kritchevsky, D., (1993). Coconut oil and sesame oil affect lymphatic absorption of cholesterol and fatty acids in rats. *J. Nutr.* 123, 1852-1858.

[45] Giovannini, I., Boldrini, G., Chiarla, C., Giuliante, F., Vellone, M., Nuzzo, G., (1999). Pathophysiologic correlates of hypocholesterolemia in critically ill surgical patients. *Intens. Care Med.* 25, 748-751.

[46] Lopez-Martinez, J., Sanchez-Castilla, M., Garcia-de-Lorenzo, A., (2000). Hypocholesterolemia in critically ill patients. *Intens. Care Med.* 26, 259-60.

[47] Bakalar, B., Zadak, Z., Pachl, J., (2001). Severe hypocholesterolemia is associated with adrenal insufficiency in multiple trauma patients. *Intens. Care Med.* 27(S2), S253.

[48] Marik, P.E., (2006). Dyslipidemia in the critically ill. *Crit. Care Clin.* 22, 151-159.

[49] USDA., (2013). USDA National Nutrient Database for Standard Reference Release 27. Available: http://ndb.nal.usda.gov/ndb/nutrients/report/nutrientsfrm?max=25&offset=0&totCount=0&nutrient1=601&nutrient2=&nutrient3=&subset=0&fg=&sort=c&measureby=m

Chapter 3

Malnutrition

Nutrition primarily deals with the components or nutrients of foods or diets to nourish the body. In other words, nutrients are those chemical compounds that are required for maintaining life activities or growing. There are two classes of nutrients in human nutrition. One class is required for the maintenance of life activities or the growth of the body, but can be produced in the human body. This group of nutrients does not have to be supplied by food intake. For example, non-essential protein amino acids belong to this group of nutrients. Another class is required for the maintenance of life activities or the growth of the body and can not be produced in the human body. This class of nutrients is defined as essential nutrients. Since essential nutrients cannot be synthesized in the human body, they must be supplied through foods or supplements. Presently, the essential nutrients identified include energy-providing compounds, essential fatty acids (linoleic acid or linolenic acid), essential amino acids (Leu, Ileu, Val, Thr, Lys, Cys + Met, Phe + Tyr, Trp, and His), vitamins (VB_1, VB_2, VB_3, VB_5, VB_6, VB_{11}, VB_{12}, VC, VA, VH, VD, VE and VK), minerals (Na, K, Mg, Ca, P, Fe, Cu, Zn, Li, Cr, Mn, Co, Se, and I; possibly including Cl, S, B, Si, F, V, Ni, Mo, and Sn). Saccharides (or named carbohydrates, mainly including starch, sucrose, lactose, maltose, glucose, galactose, fructose), triglycerides (edible fats or oils), proteins and alcohol are energy-providing compounds. However, the absence of any one of these energy-providing compounds in diets should not necessarily cause any nutritional problem in term of providing energy if the sufficient amount of the energy is supplied by others.

Malnutrition is defined as the deviation of nutrition from normal. There are two possible causes of malnutrition. One is the inadequate or excess of nutrients (e.g. energy, one or more essential nutrients) in the diets or foods. Another one is a pre-existing disease condition. This chapter is to discuss the former one, i.e. the over-intake or deficiency of certain essential nutrients that can increase the risk of CVDs. The nutrients discussed include the over-intake of calories, saturated fatty acids, iron, sodium, niacin, alcohol, saccharides, the deficiency of some B vitamins and VD as well as the over-intake or deficiency of magnesium.

Toxicity Caused by Over-intake of Calories

The over-intake of calories beyond energy expenditure causes overweight (25–<30 kg/m^2 body mass index) or obesity (body mass index ≥ 30 kg/m^2) (see Table 4 for the definition of obesity) which independently increases CVD risks. What is the mechanism of obesity caused by the over-intake of calories? How does obesity increase CVD risks? The rest context of this section is to answer these questions.

Table 4. Comparison of different methods in defining obesity

[a]BMI (kg/m^2) [1,2]	[b]WC (cm) [3,4]	[c]BFP (%) [5]	[d]WHR [6]	[e]BAI
Underweight <18.5 Healthy weight 18.5-24.9 Overweight 25.0-29.9 Obesity 30.0-39.9 Extreme obesity >40	>102 (men), >88 (women) in USA; ≥ 94 (men) and ≥ 80 (non pregnant women) in EU; >90 (South Asian and Chinese men) and > 85 (Japanese men)	>25 (men), >30 (women)	>0.9 (men), >0.85 (women)	%BFP (from dual-energy X-ray absorptiometry) = 0.93xBAI-14.89

[a]BMI: body mass index (weight/H^2) that is now routinely applied in clinical practice; limitation: unsuitable for the subject having an elevated lean body mass like athletes. [b]WC: waist circumference. [c]BFP: body fat percentage (% adioposity); limitation: difficult to measure in severely obese body due to weight limits of most equipments and insufficient diameter of CT or MRI scanners. [d]WHR: waist–hip ratio. [e]BAI: body adiposity index [(hip circumference/$height^{1.5}$)–18] [7]; limitation: being difficult to use in a clinical setting in overweight/obese postmenopausal white women [8], in severely obese women [9].

Table 5. Association of some hormones circulating levels with appetite, satiety and food intake

Hormones	Site of secretion	Fluctuation	Appetite	Satiety	Food intake	Note* [12]
ghrelin	stomach	↑ ↓	↑ ↓	↓ ↑	↓ ↑	Short-term action on the hypothalamus; Orexic effects because of possibly stimulating the release of NPY, AgRP, or orexin, and suppressing that of POMC and CRH.
CCK	small intestine	↑ ↓	↓ ↑	↑ ↓	↑ ↓	Short-term action
leptin	adipose tissue	↑ ↓	↓ ↑	↑ ↓	↑ ↓	Both short-term (12 h) or long-term (2 or 8 weeks) action on the hypothalamus; Anorexic effects because of possibly stimulating the release of CART, CRH, NT, POMC, or BDNF, and suppressing that of AgRP, orexin, GALP, Galanin, MCH, and NPY.
Insulin	β cells of pancreas	↑ ↓	↓ ↑	↑ ↓	↑ ↓	Similar to leptin that has long-term inhibitory effects on food ingestion.

*BDNF, brain-derived neurotrophic factor; NT, neurotensin; CART, cocaine- and amphetamine-regulated transcript; CRH, corticotropin-releasing hormone; NPY, neuropeptide Y; MCH, melanin concentrating hormone; AgRP, agouti-related protein; GALP, galanin, orexin and galanin-like peptide; POMC, pro-opiomelanocortin; ↑, increasing; ↓, decreasing.

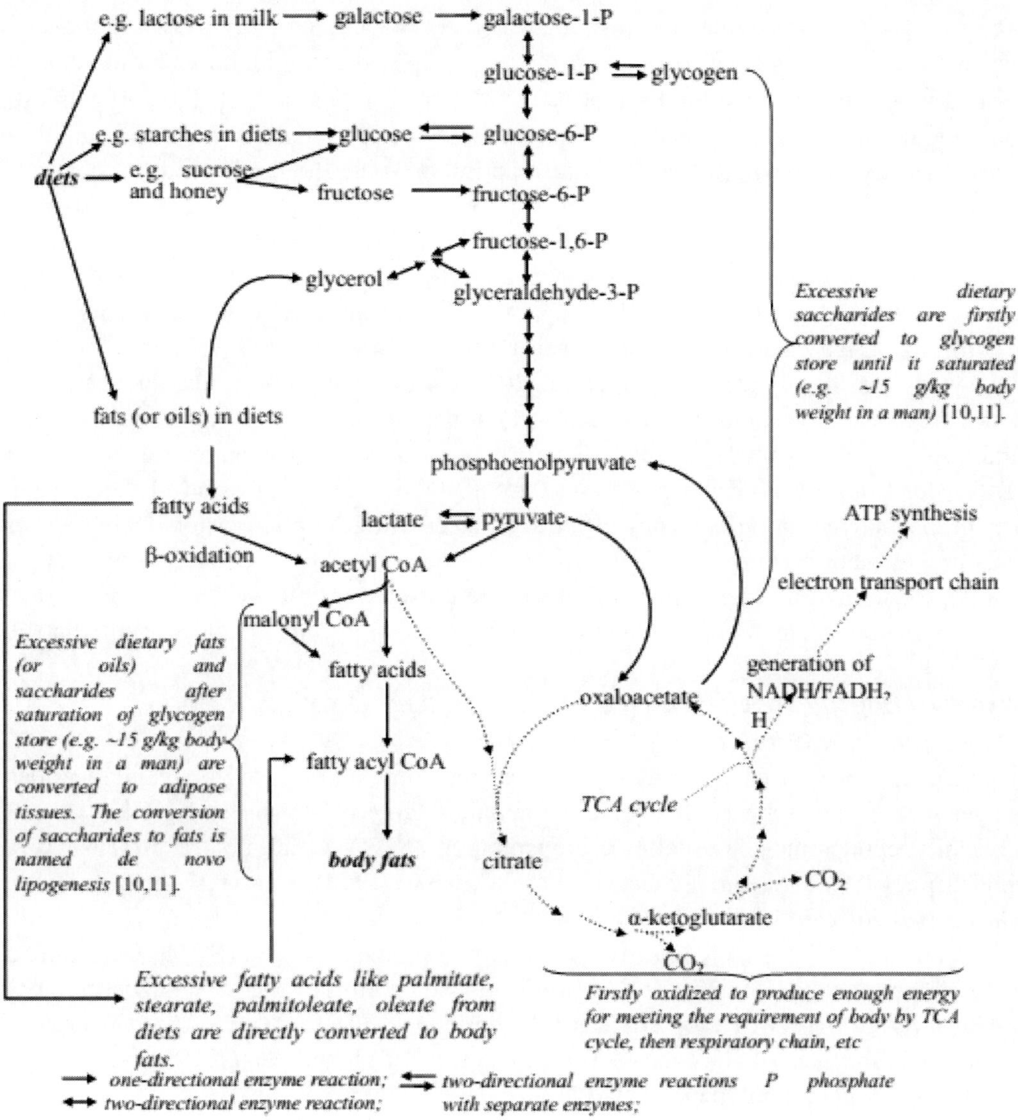

Figure 3. Pathway of converting excessive energy providing compounds to adipose tissues in the human body.

Over-intake of Calories and Obesity

Mechanism of Fat Accumulation in Adipose Tissue

The excessive body fat accumulation in adipose tissues should occur if the excessive intake of energy over its expenditure is continuously available. The excessive energy compounds that can be converted into body fats may mainly include fatty acids or glycerols from dietary fats (or oils) and monosaccharides (or those from digestible dietary polysaccharides). The pathway of converting these compounds into body fats is shown in Figure 3. Some excessive fatty acids, e.g. palmitate, stearate, palmitoleate and oleate, are directly converted to body fats (triglycerides). The excessive monosaccharides will first be stored as glycogen, whose maximum storage capacity is ~15 g/kg body weight in a man and after the saturation of the glycogen store they are disposed of by high saccharide-oxidation rates and substantial de novo lipid synthesis (~475 g saccharides converted to 150 g lipids per day) without postabsorptive hyperglycemia [10,11]. The lipid synthesis in the liver or adipose tissues normally starts with acetyl-CoA, also an intermediate in energy production pathway. The citrate in the citric acid cycle can also be reversed to acetyl-CoA, catalyzed by ATP-citrate lyase. Phosphoenolpyruvate carboxykinase catalyzes the conversion of oxaloacetate into phosphoenolpyruvate. Other enzymes required for the synthesis of triglycerides include: acetyl-CoA carboxylase for synthesizing malonyl-CoA from acetyl-CoA, fatty acid synthase for synthesizing fatty acids (e.g. palmitic acid) from malonyl-CoA and (or) acetyl-CoA, acyl-CoA synthetase for synthesizing fatty acyl-CoA from the fatty acids, elongase 6 for synthesizing stearate from palmitate, stearoyl-CoA desaturase for the reciprocal conversion of palmitoleate from stearate or oleate, and glycerol-P acyl-transferase for synthesizing triglycerides from glycerol phosphate and fatty acyl-CoA. The expression of the genes that code for the enzymes described above is up-regulated by transcription factors including sterol regulatory element-binding protein-1c, liver X receptors, carbohydrate response element binding protein, and in adipose tissues also by peroxisome proliferator activated receptor γ. Growth hormone and leptin inhibit the lipid synthesis while insulin and glucose stimulate it.

Excessive Energy Intake Caused by Imbalanced Orexigenic and Anorexigenic Compounds

The over-intake of energy may occur when the stimulation from orexigenic peptides is stronger than that from anorexigenic compounds in the human body. The identified orexigenic peptides include ghrelin, neuropeptide Y (NPY), agouti-related protein (AgRP), peptide YY (PYY), melanin-concentrating hormone (MCH), orexins (or hypocretins), galanin, β-endorphin and growth hormone-releasing hormone (GHRH). The identified anorexigenic compounds include leptin, insulin, pro-opiomelanocortin (POMC), cocaine- and amphetamine-regulated transcript (CART), melanocortins (MC), adrenocorticotropin hormone (ACTH), thyrotropin-releasing hormone (TRH), oxytocin, neurotensin, cholecystokinin (CCK), glucagon-like peptide 1 (GLP1) and 2 (GLP2), bombesin-like peptides, islet amyloid polypeptide (IAPP; also called amylin), somatostain, calcitonin-gene-related peptide, neurotensin, neuromedin U, oxyntomodulin (OXM) and glucocorticoids (e.g. cortisol in humans). The reported effect of growth hormone (GH) on food intake is still quite controversial. Experiments in non-obese and young rats implied that GH stimulated food intake [13,14] whereas a study on 8-9 weeks chicken found that GH reduced feed intake and body weight gain in a dose-dependent manner [15]. Another study on old and obese rats also indicated that GH treatment transiently reduced food intake [16].

Dietary and any other factor able to increase the effect of any orexigenic peptide (e.g. elevating its concentration or sensitivity) or decrease (or suppress) the effect of any anorexigenic peptide (e.g. lowering its concentration or sensitivity) may result in obesity. For example, an intravenous infusion or injection of ghrelin induced hunger and thus increased the food intake in healthy obese humans [17-19]. Lower serum leptin concentrations were accompanied by an increased prevalence of obesity, compared with controls [12]. Resistance (lowering sensitivity) to the anorexigenic compounds can result in obesity since some obese humans who can't be cured by leptin treatment usually have increased leptin levels in serum and adipocytes [20,21]. Defects in the downstream mediators of leptin might cause leptin resistance. Furthermore, insulin resistance (abnormally elevated insulin levels) may also induce human obesity. Improper nutrient intake, diseases, the improper use of hormonal treatment, etc could cause the imbalanced effects of orexigenic and anorexigenic compounds. Also see Table 5 for the association of circulating levels of some hormones with appetite, satiety and food intake.

Improper Nutrient Intake

An improper nutrient intake may cause anorexic hormone (e.g. leptin or insulin) resistance resulting in excessive energy intake for developing obesity. Early over-nutrition can permanently alter energy homeostasis and significantly increase leptin resistance in the arcuate nucleus, and susceptibility to obesity and insulin resistance [22].

The deficiency of some nutrients may result in imbalanced hormonal action (e.g. leptin resistance or insulin resistance) closely associated with excessive energy intake for developing obesity. The alleviation of the unpleasant experience of hunger by a high micronutrient density diet low in calories [23] may indicate that the deficiency of micronutrients could cause excessive energy intake. For example, hypovitaminosis D increased the risk of insulin resistance and the metabolic syndrome [24]. The deficiency of chromium [25], magnesium [26] or iron [27] may be closely associated with insulin resistance.

The over-intake of some nutrients may also cause anorexigenic hormonal resistance. For example, the excessive intake of Zn induced leptin resistance [28]. Reports on hyperinsulinemia, hyperglycemia and insulin resistance in mice over-expressing the selenoenzyme glutathione peroxidase 1 might indicate supranutritional selenium intake as a possible risk factor for obesity [29]. High supranutritional doses of antioxidants, e.g. administered a combination of vitamin C (1,000 mg/day) and vitamin E (400 IU/day), may be able to impair insulin sensitivity in humans [30]. Intravenous infusion of a triglyceride emulsion (1.5 ml/min) combined with heparin significantly elevated plasma free fatty acid levels (~1.8 mmol/l) in humans and induced insulin resistance [31]. The over-load of glucose in plasma may inhibit insulin action by inducing a protein kinase C-mediated serine phosphorylation of the insulin receptor in fibroblasts transfected with the human insulin receptor and therefore induce insulin resistance [32]. The over-load of amino acids, especially those branched, in plasma (~2.1 elevation) induces insulin resistance [33].

An improper portion of energy nutrients may result in leptin or insulin resistance. For example, a high-fat diet (60% kcal fat) resulted in leptin resistance after 14 days feeding whereas the corresponding control low-fat (10% kcal fat) diet did not after 28 days feeding [34]. Processed energy-dense foods were linked to insulin resistance and CVDs among Australian foragers transitioning to village life [35]. However, the type of fats or saccharides used in the diet may be the key factor for developing the hormonal resistance since a HF-Saff diet (60% kcal safflower oils, 23.8% kcal saccharides, and 16.1% kcal proteins) caused a significant elevation in serum leptin at both 2 and 4 weeks and accumulated 100 and 40% more carcass fats, respectively, compared with the Cont (11.8% kcal safflower oils, 72.1% kcal saccharides, and 16.1% kcal proteins) and HF-Fish (60% kcal fish oils, 23.8% kcal saccharides, and 16.1% kcal proteins) groups [36]. Both *in vivo* and *in vitro* studies indicated that bovine whole milk (98% of fat content being triglycerides) increased serum triglyceride and leptin levels by ~40%, which increased the risk for leptin resistance, but their free fatty acid constituents and intralipids (a source of plant triglycerides) were without effect [37].

Furthermore, a high fructose diet (60.4% kcal) resulted in leptin [38] and insulin [39] resistance while amylopectin starches promoted the development of insulin resistance in rats [40]. High meat and animal protein intakes may be associated with increased insulin resistance risks [41] whereas another study found no evidence of deleterious effects on metabolic risk factors of a substantial increase in animal proteins on the high protein diet [42]. The 7-day intervention in 8-year-old boys indicated that administrated 53 g proteins daily significantly increased fasting serum insulin levels and insulin resistance in the milk (29.4±5.1 body weight), but not in the meat (29.0±4.2 body weight), group [43]. Heat-stable lectins found in cereals might cause leptin resistance [44].

Aging

Generally, the development of obesity in the human body increases with aging. Although several other factors may also be involved in the mechanism of developing obesity, aging increased insulin resistance risks [45]. Another study indicated that aging independently increased the risk of developing leptin resistance [46].

Sleep Disturbances

Sleep disturbances, including insufficient sleep, poor sleep quality or insomnia, and obstructive sleep apnoea, might be risk factors for obesity. They may be independent risk factors for developing and exacerbating insulin resistance [47]. A single night of sleep deprivation elevated ghrelin levels that increased hunger feelings in normal-weight healthy men [48]. Recent epidemiological studies indicated that both shortened and extended sleep durations could cause increases in body weight [49].

Exposure to Traffic and Air Pollution

Some kinds of air pollution may be associated with insulin resistance. For example, it was reported that exposure to chronic traffic and air pollution may be a risk factor for the progression of insulin resistance [50]. A study on 39710-year-old children showed that traffic-related air pollution may increase the risk of insulin resistance [51].

Lesions in VHM

Lesions in the ventromedial hypothalamus (VHM) could often cause hyperphagia and consequent obesity though they increase insulin levels [52] and leptin levels [53]. One of the reasons for this may be that the production of downstream mediators, mediating the anorexigenic action of leptin, is abolished by lesions in VHM [54]. VHM lesions increase gastric emptying rate of regular diets [55], which might result from an increase in ghrelin or oxytocin levels. Furthermore, VHM lesions decrease somatostatin secretion in response to arginine stimulation [56]. Systemically administered monosodium glutamate and gold thioglucose were reported to cause VMH lesions [57].

Genetic Disorders Associated with Imbalanced Orexigenic and Anorexigenic Compounds

Such a genetic disorder as Prader-Willi syndrome can also cause obesity. People with Prader-Willi syndrome have seven genes (or some subset thereof) on chromosome 15 (q 11–13) deleted or unexpressed (chromosome 15q partial deletion) on the paternal chromosome

[58]. Abnormally the high level of ghrelin, abnormal oxytocin production and growth hormone deficiency are usually found in people with this kind of disease, which contribute to the increased appetite, hyperphagia, and obesity.

A genetically heterogeneous disorder of the primary cilium results in Bardet-Biedl syndrome associated with obesity [59]. This disease was found to be associated with leptin resistance and insulin resistance [60].

Cohen syndrome caused by a gene mutation in chromosome 8 at locus 8q22 gene COH1 [61] significantly increases the risk of obesity. This syndrome may be associated with growth hormone deficiency [62]. Other syndromes, e.g. Alström syndrome (associated with insulin resistance) [63], Turner syndrome (possibly associated with growth hormone) [64], MOMO (Macrocephaly, Obesity, Macrosomia, and Ocular anomalies with very few studies on its causes because of being a rare disorder) [65] also increase the risk of obesity, which are caused by genetic disorders.

Enterobacter

Gram-negative opportunistic pathogens in the human gut might be critical in obesity [66]. Gut microbiota may play an important role in the pathogenesis of obesity [67]. It was reported that lipopolysaccharide endotoxin produced by *Enterobacter* existing in the human gut caused obesity [68]. The induction of insulin resistance was associated with this kind of obesity [68] though further study may be necessary to the full understanding of the mechanism.

Tumors

Some types of tumers are associated with abnormal anorexic hormone levels and obesity. The ACTH-independent Cushing's syndrome is mainly caused by benign (60%) or malignant (40%) adrenal tumors [69]. Colon and breast neoplasia were found to be associated with abdominal obesity and insulin resistance [70-72].

Long Term Hormone Treatment

A long-term anorexigenic hormone treatment is very likely to cause the hormonal resistance. For example, a subsequent leptin treatment after a 21-day chronic subcutaneous leptin infusion induced leptin resistance in young lean male Long Evans rats [73,74]. The leptin treatment induced leptin resistance in aged-obese rats after 3 weeks though leptin resistance in lean rats did not occur after 4-7.5 weeks treatment [75]. A long-term insulin treatment is likely to cause insulin resistance [76]. Hyperphagia, increased weight gain, obesity, hyperinsulinemia and insulin resistance in adult life, may result from peripheral or intra-hypothalamic insulin treatments during the perinatal period [77,78]. The increased levels of intramyocellular lipids, and higher total and abdominal adipose stores were observed in the subjects with insulin resistant though they may have normal body weights [79]. The chronic administration of growth hormone in rats induced insulin resistance accompanied by decreases in insulin-stimulated autophosphorylation of insulin receptor and tyrosine phosphorylation of IRS-1 in skeletal muscles [80,81].

A long-term glucocorticoid (e.g. dexamethasone) treatment can cause insulin resistance. Cushing's syndrome (truncal obesity, relatively thin extremities, a "moon-face," and a "buffalo hump") is a condition of chronic glucocorticoid excess that may result from adrenocorticotropin hormone (ACTH)-dependent (80% cases) or –independent (20% cases;

see *Tumors*) causes endogenously [69] and the chronic administration of glucocorticoids exogenously. Increased anorexigenic ACTH or glucocorticoids levels in subjects with Cushing's syndrome may indicate that the production of downstream mediators, mediating the anorexigenic actions, is impaired. For example, glucocorticoids negatively affect the downstream action of leptin [82]. Furthermore, increased glucocorticoids decrease further activity in the hypothalamo-pituitaryadrenal axis through nongenomically mediated, direct rapid-feedback actions in the hypothalamus and pituitary [83,84].

Leptin resistance can be induced by a chronic prolactin (a single chain peptide) infusion and the administration of such a steroid hormone as progesterone [85]. These hormones may be involved in pregnancy-induced hyperphagia and subsequent obesity. Epinephrine was reported to induce insulin resistance in men [86].

Other Drugs

Glucosamine causes insulin resistance that can't be reversed by three agents (metformin, peroxovanadium and d-pinitol) known to enhance or partially mimic the effects of insulin [87]. Caffeine was reported to decrease insulin sensitivity in healthy humans, possibly as a result of elevated plasma epinephrine levels [88] while further research was suggested to be necessary [89]. High doses of rapamycin, an anti-aging drug induced insulin resistance [90]. More drugs that may induce insulin resistance have been reported in the literature, e.g. aminophylline [91], anaesthetic urethane or ketamine/xylazine [92].

Heart Transplantation

Heart transplantation might induce the development of leptin resistance and the persistence of insulin resistance [93]. The dramatic weight gain observed after heart transplantation [94] may be partly due to these impaired hormonal functions in addition to the glucocorticoid therapy.

Obesity-Associated Genotypes in Normal People

Heredity studies estimated that genetic factors contribute 45-85% of the variability in BMI [95,96] while signals from common variant loci might account for 6–11% of the genetic variation in BMI (based on an estimated heritability of 40–70%) [97]. Obesity-associated genotypes identified include ACDC (Adipocyte, C1Q and domain containing, adiponectin collagen; location: 3q27), ADRA2A (Adrenergic receptor α-2A; location: 10q24–q26), ADRA2B (Adrenergic receptor α-2B; location: 2p13–q13), ADRB1 (Adrenergic receptor β-1; location: 10q24–q26), ADRB2 (Adrenergic receptor β-2 surface; location: 5q31–q32), ADRB3 (Adrenergic receptor β-3; location: 8p12–p11.2), LEP [Leptin (obesity homologue, mouse); location 7q31.3], LEPR (Leptin receptor; location; 1p31), NR3C1 [Nuclear receptor subfamily 3, group C, member 1 (glucocorticoid receptor); location: 5q31], PPARG (Peroxisome proliferative activated receptor, γ; location: 3p25), UCP1 [Uncoupling protein 1 (mitochondrial, proton carrier); location: 4q28–q31], UCP2 [Uncoupling protein 2 (mitochondrial, proton carrier); location: 11q13] and UCP3 [Uncoupling protein 3 (mitochondrial, proton carrier); location: 11q13] [98].

Excessive Energy Intake Caused by Impairments in Neurotransmitters

Dopaminergic pathways modulate neuronal systems related to reward sensitivity, incentive motivation, conditioning, self-control, stress reactivity and interoceptive awareness [99]. Impairments in dopaminergic pathways are usually associated with excessive food intake. Drugs decreasing the activity of dopamine (DA) D2 receptors increase food intake and cause significant weight gain. In this case, it is likely to see an increase in DA levels in the human body. For example, a transgenic mouse with persistently elevated striatal DA increased food intake and increased incentive motivation to consume foods [100]. Conversely, drugs able to elevate brain DA level are anorexigenic. DA agonists normalize the body weight of genetically obese mice. Reports on the lower extracellular DA and amphetamine-induced DA release in obese rats due to a cafeteria diet were found in the literature [101] though animals whose DA system in the ventral tegmental area was rendered inactive did not seek food, and starved to death if left to themselves, but they consumed foods that were placed in their mouths and showed facial expressions indicative of pleasure [102]. Therefore, decreases in DA signaling in striatal regions [decreases in DA D2 (D2R) receptors (perhaps increase in DA levels in the body) and in DA release] are associated with reward (nucleus accumbens) but also with habits and routines (dorsal striatum) in obesity.

Such neurotransmitters as opioid, cannabinoid, gamma-aminobutyric acid, among others appear to be associated with the hedonic ('liking') response to foods [103]. For example, endogenous opioids are facilitators of sweet or fat tastants intake [104] while binge eating disorders link to the functional A118G polymorphism of the mu-opioid receptor gene [105].

Obesity Caused by Decreased Energy Expenditure

Decreased Basal Metabolic Rate (BMR)

Basal metabolism (BM) consumes about three-quarters of body's requirements for energy used for maintaining body temperature and biochemical processes, heartbeat, and respiration. The energy expenditure of BM expressed as BMR is usually measured by lying down in a warm room after eating for 12 h and at complete physical and mental rest.

Several factors can decrease BMR. Increase in age tends to decrease BMR. Short-term weight loss by very-low-calorie diets significantly reduced fat-free mass with a concomitant decrease in absolute BMR [106]. The extent of decreases in BMR may be associated with dietary composition. For example, the decrease in BMR was the greatest with the low-fat diet, intermediate with the low–glycemic index diet, and the least with the very low-carbohydrate diet [107]. People living in very hot climates may decrease their BMR by about 9.9% compared to cooler climates. Fasting and low body weight can also reduce BMR. Other factors reported to induce decreases in energy expenditure include osteocalcin knockout [108], prolonged sub-maximal exercise in a warm environment [109], an oral intake of some drugs e.g. clonidine [110] or glutamine [111], some diseases e.g. Prader-Willi syndrome [112] or hypothyroidism [113], sex steroid deficiency [114], prenatal high protein exposure [115], the infusion of some hormones such as melanin concentrating hormone [116], acute sleep deprivation [117], losses in skeletal muscle mass (associated with such factors as aging, sedentary lifestyle) [118], etc. Reports on the effects of sexes and ages on BMR appear to be controversial. It was reported that BMR decreased with aging and might decrease in women

[119] whereas no effect of sex and age on BMR independent of body size, body composition and activity were reported [120].

Decreased Adaptive Thermogenesis (AT)

AT (or called *Diet-induced thermogenesis*) is the phenomenon of an increase in heat production by the body after foods are ingested. AT may partly result from the digestive processes in the digestive tract and partly from the metabolism of absorbed foods in the body.

AT might be multicausal. Depending upon the proportion of proteins, saccharides and fats in mixed diets, the amount of heat produced by AT is about 5-15% of the energy value of the daily foods ingested [121]. The ingestion of saccharides and fats can cause less increase in heat production than that of pure proteins. It is also suggested that a sedentary lifestyle may have a less AT in males, compared to an active lifestyle [122].

Decreased Physical Activity

Physical activity is a more variable factor that affects overall energy expenditure than BM and AT. The duration and intensity of the activity as well as body size determine the amount of energy consumed. Normally, the physical activity with shorter time, or less intensity expends less energy than that with longer time or more intensity, respectively. Other effects of decreased the physical activity are described above in BMR and AT.

Excessive Energy Intake and Decreased Expenditure Caused by Misaligned Eating Time

Nocturnal mice fed only during the 12-h light phase tend to intake more energy, be less active and gain more weight than those fed only during 12-h dark phase [123], which also causes a decrease in dark phase body temperature [124]. The mechanism of this phenomenon may be mainly associated with the adaptability of body to store the excessive energy ingested (small amount of energy needed because of sleeping shortly after eating during the light phase) for supporting locomotive activity during the dark phase. Metabolic processes (including changes in hormones, neurotransmitters, some enzymes, fat deposition, etc) may adjust to synchronize with the change in food intake time so that a new energy homeostasis and body weight, etc are established. Conversely, human is usually diurnal, who is easy to get night eating syndrome (severe obesity) [125].

Excessive Energy Intake and Decreased Energy Expenditure Caused by Neonatal Nicotine Exposure

Neonatal nicotine exposure may induce leptin resistance and decrease energy expenditure in childhood and adulthood. Maternal smoking during pregnancy might increase the risk of childhood obesity [126,127]. The increased adiposity in the offspring might be associated with nicotine exposure, the main addictive compound of tobacco smoke, in gestational and lactation periods [128-131]. Lactation may be a crucial period for programming later obesity by nicotine, with thyroid dysfunction, a possible contributing factor, since a maternal nicotine exposure only during lactation induces overweight, higher central adiposity, hyperleptinemia, leptin and insulin resistance, and secondary hypothyroidism in adult rat offspring [104].

Energy Density of a Meal

The intake of high energy density foods is very easy to cause excessive energy intake. Increase in the proportion of fats (9 kcal/g) in a meal elevates its energy density. Increase in the proportion of non-energy components (e.g. dietary fibers) decreases the energy density of a meal, compared to that with higher proportion of saccharides (4 kcal/g) and proteins (4 kcal/g). Alcoholism (7 kcal/g) that might decrease the consumption of starches or proteins may also increase the energy density of a meal.

Conclusion

Body fat accumulation in adipose tissues mainly caused by excessive energy intake over its expenditure is associated with obesity. This could result from an excessive food intake, or decrease in energy expenditure, or the combined effect of both factors. Such factors as impaired neurogenic activities (neurotransmitter level), hormonal and enzymatic systems, genetic determinants or disorders, the improper digestive enzyme activities of energy components, the properties of foods, or other occasional diseases [e.g. lesions in the ventromedial hypothalamus, gut microorganisms (e.g. *Enterobacter*), Cushing's syndrome] may be involved in an excessive food intake. Factors that decrease energy expenditure might include osteocalcin knockout, prolonged sub-maximal exercise in a warm environment, an oral intake of some drugs such as clonidine or glutamine, some diseases (e.g. Prader-Willi syndrome or hypothyroidism), sex steroid deficiency, prenatal high protein exposure, the infusion of some hormones such as melanin concentrating hormone, acute sleep deprivation, losses in skeletal muscle mass, dietary composition, decreased physical activities, etc. Misaligned eating time and neonatal nicotine exposure might be associated with an excessive energy intake and decreased energy expenditure. Meal energy density is also involved in an excessive energy intake.

Obesity and CVDs

Obesity or overweight may result in hyperlipidemia with increased blood LDLCs and VLDLCs, decreased blood HDLCs (i.e. a decreased HDLC/LDLC ratio), and elevate blood viscosity [132] up to the level higher than normal (3×10^{-3} to 4×10^{-3} Pa.s). These and other obesity-associated factors such as, the function of adipose tissue derivatives (adipokines and cytokines), neurohumoral pathways, metabolic functions, the modulation of pressor/depressor mechanisms, diabetes (insulin resistance), and leptin resistance, may induce hypertension or CVDs [133] (also see Figure 4).

Hyperlipidemia is primarily concerned with increases in the level of fasting TCs (>200 mg/dL) or LDLCs (>130 mg/dL) in blood, which may or may not link with increased level (>150 mg/dL) of total triglycerides [134]. Hyperlipidemia with a decreased HDLC/TC or

LDLC ratio is a well predictor of developing CVDs, which has been discussed in the section entitled "Biochemical Marks of CVDs" in Chapter 1 and the section entitled "Dietary Cholesterol and Risk of CVDs" in Chapter 2.

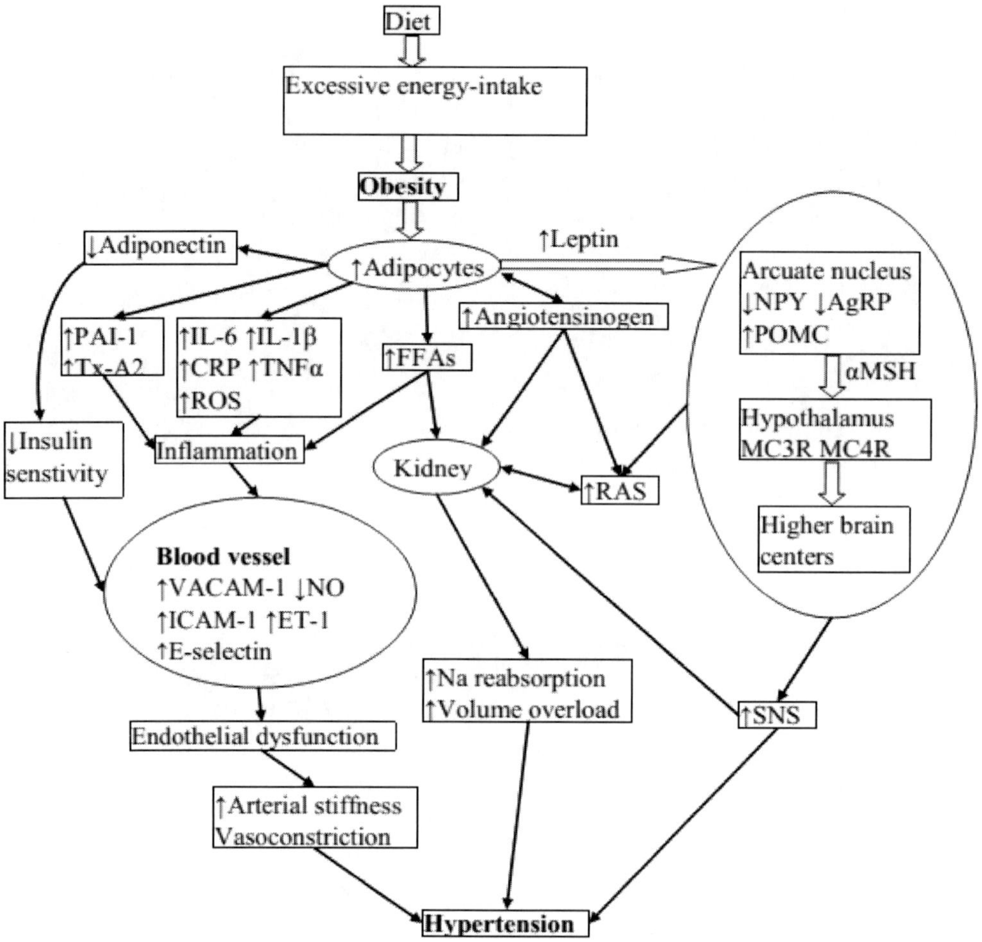

Figure 4. Mechanisms of hypertension associated with obesity. ↑, increase; ↓, decrease; NPY, neuropeptide Y; POMC, pro-opiomelanocortin; a-MSH, a-melanocyte-stimulating hormone; MC3R, melanocortin 3 receptor; MC4R, melanocortin 4 receptor; PAI-1, plasminogen activator inhibitor-1; Tx-A2, thromboxane A2; IL-6, interleukin-6; IL-1β, interleukin-1β; TNFα, tumor necrosis factor-α; CRP, C-reactive protein; ROS, reactive oxygen species; FFAs, free fatty acids; VCAM-1, vascular cell adhesion molecule-1; ICAM-1, inter-cellular adhesion molecule-1; NO, nitric oxide; ET-1, endothelin-1; RAS, rennin–angiotensin system; SNS, sympathetic nervous system; AgRP, agouti-related peptide [133].

The viscosity of blood is a measure of its resistance to flow in vessels or to gradual deformation by tensile or shear stress. It is mainly determined on aggregation (in low flow/shear conditions) or deformation (in high flow/shear conditions) of red cells, plasma viscosity mainly depending upon lipoproteins, reactant globulins, plasma fibrinogen, and the volume fraction of haematocrit (red blood cells) [135,136]. Many scientific evidences indicate that an elevated blood viscosity may be a risk factor for CVDs [137-139].

Adiponectin is a protein encoded by ADIPOQ gene. It is associated with the regulation of glucose concentration and the breakdown of fatty acids. It may be involved in suppressing metabolic derangements of causing atherosclerosis, or type 2 diabetes. Therefore, the decreased adiponectin caused by obesity may increase the risk of atherosclerosis, or type 2 diabetes. Decrease in insulin activity caused by decreased adiponectin as well as increased inflammation (caused by increased PAI-1, Tx-A2, IL-6, IL-1β, CRP, TNFα, ROS and FFAs that result from obesity) may result in increases in VACAM-1, ICAM-1, ET-1 and E-selectin as well as a decrease in NO that acts as a vascular homeostatic agent and vasodilator. This would cause endothelial dysfunction that subsequently result in the increase in arterial stiffness. The increased FFAs and angiotensinogen caused by obesity may also increase Na reabsorption and volume overload in kidneys and subsequently result in hypertension. Obesity can cause an decrease in leptin activities and therefore increase leptin levels in blood. The increased leptin level may cause an increase in POMC and decrease in NPY and AgRP that result in an increase in SNS. An increase in SNS can directly cause hypertension or an increase in Na reabsorption and volume overload in kidneys, which also causes hypertension.

However, there is also a controversial report that states a positive association of high (except for low) molecular weight adiponectin with coronary artery diseases (140). This may indicate that other collaboration factors may also exist and should not be ignored.

Toxicity Caused by Over-Intake of Saturated Fatty Acids

Dietary Sources of Saturated Fatty Acids

The saturated fatty acids (SFAs) discussed in this section refer to those that partially comprise fats or oils (i.e. triglycerides) in diets or foods. Like every other fatty acid, different SFAs contain different numbers of carbon atoms. The number of their carbon atoms is mainly 4 - 20. SFAs are usually classed as three groups according to the number of carbon atoms. One is named short chain saturated fatty acids (SCFAs) that contain <6 carbon atoms. Those containing 6-10 carbon atoms are named medium chain fatty acids (MCFAs). Those containing 12 to 18 carbon atoms or more are named long chain saturated fatty acids (LCFAs).

Table 6. Typical SFA contents (g/100 g) of some edible oils and fats

Oils	SFA Content	Fats	SFA Content
Coconut oil	86.6	Water buffalo's milk fat	64.2
Palm kernel oil	81.6	Goat's milk fat	63.6
Palm oil	49.4	Cow's milk fat	63.5
Olive oil	13.7	Cocoa butter	59.6
Low-erucic rapeseed oil	7.5	Lamb suet	59.7
High-linoleic acid sunflower oil	10.4	Lard	45.0
Soybean oil	15.4	Beef suet	46.0
Corn oil	12.8	Horse suet	35.6

However, some scientists may denote those having 12 carbon atoms (e.g. lauric acid) as a LCFA. SCFAs (mainly butyric acid) are normally found in milk fats. SCFAs with <4 carbon atoms are unlikely to be found in other dietary fats or oils, including those originated from plants or animals. Stearic acid (18:0), palmitic acid (16:0), myristic acid (14:0), and lauric acid (12:0) are the predominant SFAs in the diets or foods. SFAs mainly exist in animal or some plant (such as cocoa) fats. Typical SFA contents of some edible oils and fats are shown in Table 6.

Over-Intake of Saturated Fatty Acids and CVDs

The over-intake of saturated fatty acids (SFAs) may be involved in developing plaque and thrombus [141,142]. SFAs elevate LDLCs in humans [143]. The CVD risk of energy-providing nutrients, in order, was reported to be as the following: SFAs > carbohydrates (19.4 and 29.2% of total energy contributed by sugars and starches, respectively) > monounsaturated fats > polyunsaturated fats [144] while the CVD risk of unsaturated fatty acids, in order, may be as the following: ω-9 > ω-6 (mainly linoleic acid, having 2 double bonds) > ω-3 (mainly linolenic acid, having 3 double bonds) fatty acids [145,146].

The mechanism of SFAs intake being associated with the increased risk of CVDs, compared with unsaturated fatty acids, may mainly involve the induction of inflammation (the activation of NF-κB, increased CRP, the expression of Cox2 and other inflammatory markers such as IL-6 and TNF-α), endothelial dysfunction (increased SICAM, SVCAM, and E-selectin), and the elevation of clot formation (increased coagulant activity of factor VII). Other factors such as the induction of hyperinsulinemia may also be involved.

The risk of over-intake of SFAs for CVDs might be counteracted by other dietary factors, since the "French paradox" does exist (higher intake of SFAs with lower prevalence of CVDs in France than in some other European countries) [147]. The beneficial dietary factors in France may include: significant amount of red wine drinking that contains resveratrol and other polyphenolic compounds, lower obesity rates in France than in most other European countries, and significantly higher vegetable and fruit consumption.

Dietary Recommendations for SFAs Intake

The WHO and the US Dietary Guidelines recommend <10% of total energy intake from SFAs. However,the American Heart Association guidelines suggest <7% [148] though theω-6 (linoleic acid)/ω-3 (linolenic acid) ratio of unsaturated fatty acids in daily diets may also be a vital factor (4 to 1 or lower suggested to be optimal)[146].

SFAs can be synthesized in the human body though the extent is quite low and may not be required in the diets. And also, many scientific evidences tend to indicate an positive association of SFAs with the risk of CVDs. Therefore, it is suggested that the intake of SFAs be as low as possible [149]. The establishment of nutrient goals or recommendations should consider the SFAs intake being limited. The ESFA [149] also suggested that Adequate Intake, Lower Threshold Intake, Average Requirement, or no Population Reference Intake be set.

It should be noted that the recommendation for the appropriate amount of intake of butyric acid may not be the same as that for other SFAs since butyrate was reported to be capable of greatly enhancing the efficiency of induced pluripotent stem cell derivation from human adult or fetal fibroblasts [150]. Therefore, more research work may be necessary for the evaluation of the dietary safety and biological function of butyric acid and recommendation for its safe intake.

Toxicity Caused by Over-Intake of Iron

Dietary Iron and Human Nutrition

Iron is an essential mineral for human life. It is required for constituting an erythrocyte protein (hemoglobin) that is responsible for transporting oxygen in the lungs to the tissues. It also plays a role in metabolism since it partially comprises myoglobin that supplies oxygen to muscles. It is essential for the function of normal cells, development, growth, and the production of connective tissue or some hormones. The majority of elemental irons (3-4 g) in an adult's body is in the form of hemoglobin [151]. The rest of irons is mainly for comprising ferritin or hemosiderin (degraded ferritin) in the bone marrow, spleen, and liver or for constituting myoglobin in muscle tissues. The absorption and distribution of irons in the human body is mainly regulated by a circulating peptide hormone (hepcidin) [152].

It must be supplied by eating foods or drinking beverages. In other words, daily diets should be the predominant source of dietary irons except for a pharmaceutic supplement. Dietary irons may be classified as nonheme and heme (iron combined with protoporphyrin IX). There are only nonheme irons in plant or some iron-fortified foods. Both nonheme irons and heme irons are present in animal products such as poultry, seafoods, and other meats. Heme irons account for ca. 10% to 15% of total iron intakes in western populations [153].

Only small quantities of irons absorbed by the human body lose with feces and urine. Some losses take place in the skin and the gastrointestinal tract. Menstruating women usually lose significant amount of irons with blood losses.

Iron is found in a variety of foods. Its content is very high in some foods, such as 445.5 mg/kg in raw beef spleen, 418.9 mg/kg in raw lamb spleen, 223.2 mg/kg in raw pork spleen, and 233.0 mg/kg in raw pork liver [154]. Compared with the tolerable upper intake level (45 mg/day) recommended [155], most foods should be safe for consumption for healthy individuals, but those foods with the top range of the iron content described above and any canned food or drink in a poorly tinned can could be dangerous.

Over-Intake of Iron and CVDs

The over-intake of irons increases CVD risks [156]. For nomal healthy people and those with primary hemochromatosis caused by genetical mutation, the harmful level of iron intake is greatly different.

People with hemochromatosis (an illness resulted from hemochromatosis (HFE) gene mutation) usually develop an overload of irons in the body [158]. In whites population, 4.4/1000 are homozygous for the HFE gene mutation and develop hemochromatosis though ca. 10% of the population carry the most common mutation gene (C282Y) [159]. Other ethnic people do not commonly develop this disease. Signs of iron toxicity are usually observed in individuals with hereditary hemochromatosis at the age of 30 years if no treatment is previously undertaken [160]. The symptoms of iron toxicity include heart disease, impaired pancreatic function, hepatocellular carcinoma, and liver cirrhosis. The presence of certain amount of irons and vitamin C in diets or supplements was reported to be harmful for treating hereditary hemochromatosis [158].

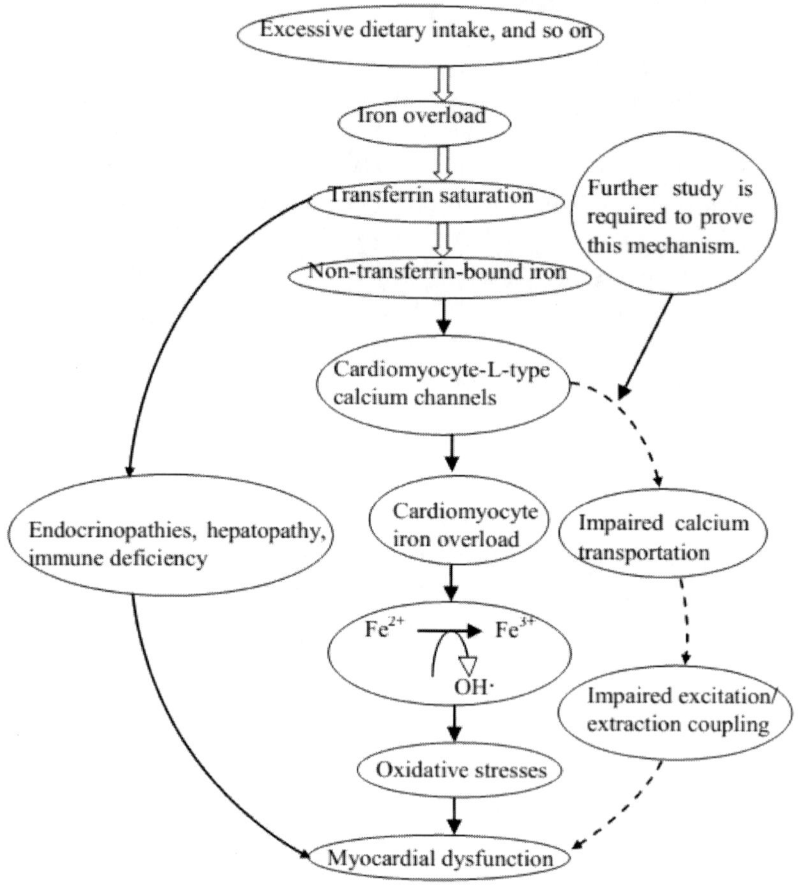

Figure 5. Mechanism of myocardial dysfunction associated with iron overload. This figure is developed on the basis of data by Kremastinos and Farmakis [157].

Apart from increased iron absorption or accumulation due to primary hemochromatosis and ineffective erythropoiesis, which is caused by hemoglobinopathies, melodysplastic syndromes, and repetitive transfusions, an excessive dietary intake can also result in iron overload and can cause myocardial dysfunction [157]. The harmful level of irons in blood was reported to be serum ferritin >300 ng/mL that is associated with cardiac symptoms [157]. Figure 5 indicates the suggested mechanism of iron toxicity. The daily intake of >50 mg elemental irons in adults may be chronically toxic with significant gastrointestinal symptoms, myocardial symptoms, and even diabetes, but the acute toxicity caused by oral doses below about 10-20 mg/kg body weight has not been reported [161].

Toxicity Caused by Over-Intake of Sodium

Sodium is essentially required for proper life activities in the body. It is vital for controlling blood volume or blood pressure in the body. The proper function of nerves (e.g. the transmission of nerve impulses) and muscles (e.g. relaxation or contraction) also needs the help of sodium. Therefore, sodium is regarded as an essential nutrient. It has to be supplied by eating foods or drinking beverages. These mean that the daily intake of sodium throughout lifetime is necessary. What is its occurrence in daily diets and dietary safety?

Dietary Sodium

Most natural staple foods contain sodium. There is also sodium in other natural foods, for example celery and other vegetables, beets, and milk. Sodium exists in drinking water, but its concentration is dependent upon the source.

In food industries, sodium-containing ingredients are often added. Sodium benzoate, baking soda (sodium bicarbonate), sodium saccharin, sodium nitrite, and monosodium glutamate are quite commonly added in some food products. Such seasonings as bouillon cubes, garlic salt, onion salt, soy sauce, Worcestershire sauce may contain the sodium-containing ingredients mentioned above. Generally, sodium is very high in most snack foods. Sodium-containing ingredients are usually added to such processed products as vegetables, canned soups, and meats (e.g. ham, sausage or bacon).

Sodium chlodride (table salt) is the most common form of salt. It is daily used for cooking or stir-frying vegetables, meats, etc.

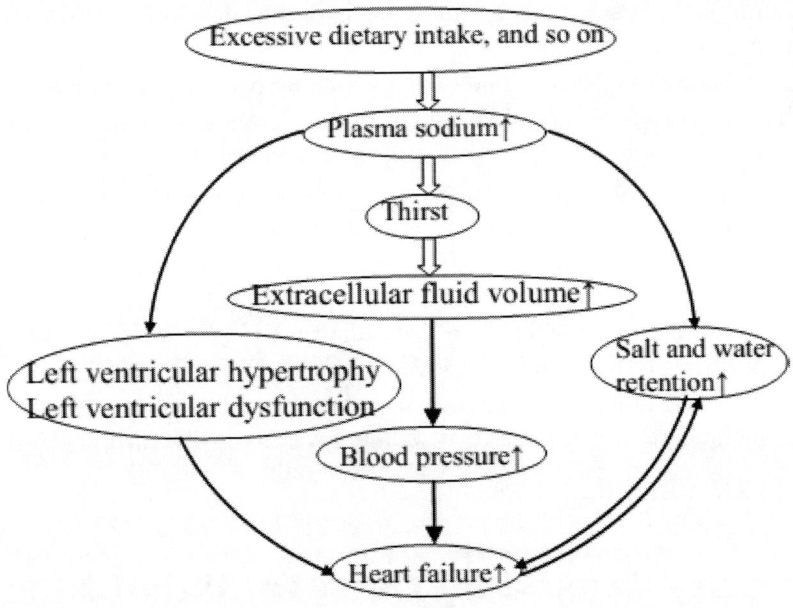

Figure 6. Mechanism of heart failure associated with sodium overload. This figure is developed on the basis of data by He and others [162] and De Wardener and others [175].

Over-Intake of Sodium and CVDs

Although sodium is essential, too much of it just like any other nutrients is bad, including salt (sodium chloride). The over-intake of sodium may increase the risk of damaging the cardiovascular system (CVS) [162]. The kidneys could be overwhelmed by the excessive amount of sodium chloride so that they become incapable of excreting it properly, resulting in the accumulation of it in the blood. The serious consequence of this reaction is further to induce high blood pressure (or called hypertension) that consecutively has the potential of inducing life-threatening CVDs (e.g. strokes or heart attacks).

The adverse effects of a high salt intake on the cardiovascular system may include: 1, elevating blood pressure [163,164]; 2, increasing the mass of left ventricular (LV) wall (LV hypertrophy) [165]; 3, inducing LV dysfunction [165]; 4, stiffening conduit vessels [166]; 5, thickening and narrowing resistance vessels [167]; 6, subsequently increasing the risk of strokes and heart failure [162]; 7, directly increasing the incidence of acutely decompensated heart failure (≥2.8 g Na/day) [168]; 8, playing a key role as an effect modifier in blood pressure genetics [169]; 9, worsening such a CVD as myocardial infarction (also see Figure 6). It was also reported that >3634 mg/L Na in the blood is defined as hypernatremia [170] and >4140 mg/L would increase the mortality of CVDs [171]. The recommended intake of sodium is <2.3 g/day in the USA where 1 in 3 adults has one or more types of CVDs [172-174].

The adverse effect of a high sodium intake on the cardiovascular system may also vary with age, genes, and such other factors as gender and body weight. In contrast to individuals over 30 years of age, the blood pressure in young men <26 years does not increase with an increase in a salt intake [175]. Salt-sensitive individuals (about 40-50% of all patients with hypertension [176]) develop hypertension on a high-sodium intake, but remain normotensive on a low-sodium intake, while resistant individuals do not develop hypertension on a high-sodium intake [175].

In case of established CVDs, a study on 3681 participants predicted that the death rates decreased across increasing tertiles of 24-hour sodium excretion (regarded as an indicator of a sodium intake), namely 4.1% in the low (2.46 g), 1.9% in the medium (3.86 g), and 0.8% in the high excretion group (5.98 g) [177], whereas some experts criticized that this study was weak, the study being small with low event rates and relatively young participants [178]. Other studies supported this conclusion. For example, the sodium reduction was reported to have a harmful effect on patients with established heart failure (2.30–5.75 g/d intake compared with 1.61–2.00 g/d intake) [179] and diabetes (24-h urinary sodium excretion of <102 mmol/day compared with that of >102 mmol/day) [180]. This might be partly due to that patients with heart failure may develop hyponatremia (the failure of kidneys to excrete sodium free urine in order to keep a normal sodium level in the blood while the sodium intake is not enough).

Toxicity Caused by Over-Intake of Niacin

Niacin is a B vitamin that is soluble in water, which is given a number as vitamin B_3 [181]. It is the collective name of nicotinic acid and its derivative (amide), i.e. nicotinamide.

The nicotinamide comprises the essential part of coenzymes, i.e. nicotinamide adenine dinucleotide (NAD) and nicotinamide adenine dinucleotide phosphate (NADP). NAD and NADP are involved in oxidation-reduction (redox) reactions (e.g. the key metabolic pathway of respiration - the Krebs cycle reactions) that are associated with the transfer of electrons. They are required by as many as 200 enzymes. The reactions of producing energy need NAD, which destructures fats, carbohydrates, alcohol and proteins (usually defined as catabolism). The reactions of biosynthesis (anabolism) also need NADP, which isinvolved in the production of all macromolecules, including cholesterols and fatty acids [182]. NAD is also involved in non-redox reactions. For example, it is the substrate for two enzymes (poly-ADP-ribose polymerase and mono-ADP-ribosyltransferases) [182]. Therefore, niacin is an essential nutrient for human life since it can not be produced in the body. It can only be supplied by eating foods or drinking beverages. These mean that the daily intake of niacin throughout lifetime is necessary. What is its occurrence in our daily diets and dietary safety?

Dietary Niacin

The recommended daily allowance of niacin in USA is 2–12, 14, 16, and 18 mg for children, women, men, and pregnant or breast-feeding women, respectively, while 35 mg/day are suggested to be its tolerable upper intake levels for adult men and women [183].

Niacin is found in most natural foods. It is very rich in meats, the animal liver, peanuts, and wheat bran. For example, its content is 153.0 mg/kg in raw pork liver, 159.3 mg/kg in Spanish peanuts, and 270.0 mg/kg in defatted peanuts [154]. We should be aware of the potential toxicity of long term consumption of the foods with so high content of niacin just mentioned above, especially for children.

However, a study on patients with dyslipoproteinemia (or an atherosclerotic CVD) indicated that extended-release niacin, 1500 to 2000 mg per day improved HDLC and triglyceride levels [184]. Furthermore, the treatment of some CVDs with niacin (1000 – 2000 mg/day) was suggested [185,186]. Others approved this conclusion [181]. These doses that are supposed to be effective on treating CVDs are much higher than the tolerable upper intake levels of niacin recommended by FNBIM [183]. Normal daily diets are very unlikely to provide so high level of niacin. They may only be achieved by an artificial supplementation. The safety of so high level of niacin intake throughout lifetime needs to be carefully evaluated.

It seems that no report on the ability of appropriate amount (especially that can be achieved by daily dietary practice) of niacin intake to prevent CVDs can be found in the past literature. It would be worth carrying out this kind of scientific study.

Over-Intake of Niacin and CVDs

The over-intake of niacin was reported to cause cardiac arrhythmias [187] and other problems, which could be deadly in some cases [188]. An intake of niacin ≥1,000 mg/day caused a substantial increase in blood homocysteine [189]. Furthermore, it was reported that 1.5 g of nicotinic acid intake three times for 8 weeks was found to be associated with hyperglycemia and hyperuricemia that are risk factors for CVDs [190]. However, these levels of niacin are not likely with usual dietary practices.

On the other hand, the discontinuation of this kind of treatment was recommended [191]. Therefore, further precise toxicological and effective studies may be necessary for resolving the dispute.

Toxicity Caused by Over-Intake of Alcohol

Dietary alcohol refers to ethyl alcohol (or named ethanol). It is an energy-providing compound, 1 g of which can provide 7 kcal calories. Its molecular formula is CH_3-CH_2-OH. This compound is a liquid that is flammable, volatile and colorless, having a strong chemical odor.

This compound is edible. Therefore, it is commonly consumed by significant number of people in the world. What is its occurrence in diets? How does it affect human's health, especially the health of the cardiovascular system?

Alcohol in Diets

The presence of ethyl ethanol in overripe fruits is quite common. It is not commonly found in natural staple foods, most other foods, vegetables, and most ripe fruits. Edible ethyl ethanol is artificially produced by fermenting sugars by yeast. It is usually processed into alcohol beverages, such as wine, red wine, beer, and champagne.

It has been reported that ca. 2 billion people drink alcoholic beverages worldwide [192]. The level of alcohol consumption may be classified as the following: high (more than 3 drinks/day for men and more than 2 drinks/day for women), moderate (up to 3 drinks/day (i.e. 1–21 drinks/week) for men and up to 2 drinks/day (i.e. 1–14 drinks/week) for women), and low (less than 1 drink/week, reference category) [193]. A drink may be defined as a shot of hard liquor (45 mL), or a standard glass of wine (150 mL) or beer (355 mL) [194].

Over-Intake of Alcohol and CVDs

The over-intake of alcohol increases CVD risks though low to moderate alcohol consumption may lower it. For example, it was reported that children or alcohol-naïve adults may experience an increased blood pressure, heart rate, etc even at less than 100 mg/dL ethanol in the blood [195]. A dosage in excess of 50 g/day was considered to be a risk for coronary heart disease (CHD) [196], while others reported that a daily consumption of >80 g/day is harmful [197]. Furthermore, most reported alcoholic patients with detectable changes in cardiac structure and function consumed >90 g/day of alcohol for at least 5 years [198-201].

The toxic dosage of alcohol may vary with the presence of other components in diets, ages, gender, genes, and health status. For example, one study concluded that the harmful dosage of alcohol was 52 g/day for females and 114 g/day for males [202]. In patients with established CVDs or diabetes, an ingestion of 1.25 g/kg/day was reported to be harmful [203]. The risk of alcoholic cardiomyopathy and myopathy is greater in women than in men [204]. Genetic predisposition (HLA-B8, alcohol dehydrogenase alleles) and such environmental factors as cobalt and arsenic were suggested to be involved in the etio-pathogenesis of alcoholic heart diseases [205].

The mechanism of alcoholic CVDs may involve atrial fibrillation, cardiomyopathy, an increased thickening and scarring of cardiac connective tissues, altered oxidative stress, induced electrolyte imbalance, and negative inotropic effects through calcium channel inhibition in ventricular cells [194]. The changes in cardiac metabolism in myocardial failure and after alcohol intake have been discussed in the literature [206]. And also, the calory content of alcohol is much higher than that of proteins and energy-providing saccharides. Therefore, large amounts of alcohol intake may result in obesity that is a risk factor of CVDs (see the section entitled "Toxicity Caused by Over-intake of Calories" of this chapter).

Toxicity Caused by Over-Intake of Saccharides

Saccharides are also named carbohydrates. Some of them are energy-providing compounds, 1 g of which can supply 4 kcal calories. The energy-providing saccharides are digestible, including starches and sugars (e.g. sucrose, maltose, lactose) or absorbable (e.g. glucose, fructose, galactose). Some others, for example dietary fibers (including soluble and insoluble fibers), are not digestible and therefore can supply very few energy to the human body. These saccharides may be positively or negatively associated with CVD risks depending on the amount of intake, glycemic index or load, body condition (e.g. obesity), etc.

Dietary Sources of Saccharides

Dietary saccharides are primarily originated from plant food resources. Some of them are staple foods in many countries, e.g. starchy foods in Asia and Africa. Some of them are not staple foods, but widely used as food additives in many kinds of processed foods, such as sugars, polysaccharide gels.

Dietary fibers widely exist in plant foods, such as vegetables, edible roots or tubers, grains, and fruits. Some beverages (or soups or ice cream or yogurt) usually contain artificially added soluble fibers, such as sodium carboxymethyl cellulose, pectin.

Starches are the main micronutrient in grains (e.g. rice, corn, wheat), some tubers (e.g. potatoes), some roots (e.g. sweet potatoes, cassava), and some tree stems (e.g. sago palm). The edible part of these plants usually contain more than 70% starches by a dry weight. Starches are also rich in peas (e.g. cow or chickpeas) and beans (e.g. mung, lentils or favas beans). There are also other starchy food resources, e.g. yams, water chestnuts, chestnuts, taro, rye, sorghum, Polynesian arrowroot, oats, millet, malanga, katakuri, kudzu, colacasia, canna, buckwheat, breadfruit, barley, bananas, arracacha, arrowroot and acorns.

Sugars are mainly employed as sweeteners in processing snack foods or beverages and cooking. Sucrose is usually produced by extracting it from sugar canes or beets or palms. Maltose and glucose are usually made by hydrolyzing starches. High fructose syrup is also produced by hydrolyzing starches followed by an enzymatic conversion of some glucoses into fructoses. Lactose is isolated from milk. The main components of honey are glucose and fructose.

Over-Intake of Saccharides and CVDs

The association of increased dietary fibers intake with decreased ischaemic heart diseases was suggested in the 1970s [207]. Since then, many observational or experimental investigations into the association of fiber rich foods or dietary fibers with decreased CVD risk factors (e.g. plasma cholesterols, insulin sensitivity, central obesity, or hypertension) or total CVD risks have been reported [208,209]. The negative association of dietary fibers with CVD risks may result from their biological effect on individual risk factor, which may involve in many mechanisms. The elevation of postprandial blood lipid or glucose can be alleviated by viscous and soluble fibers that can form gels of being able to slow the absorption of lipid or glucose from the small intestine [210,211]. These authors also stated that the speed of gastric emptying can be slowed by the gels formed, which can maintain satiety and therefore result in less energy intake and prevent obesity or overweight. The additional fermentation of resistant starches or soluble fibers by bacteria in the large intestine can produce SCFs that are helpful for decreasing the circulating levels of cholesterols [212].

The association of starch intake with CVD risks is largely dependent upon the glycemic index (GI) or load (GL). Generally, a starch that has a higher GI or GL results in a higher CVD risk. The GI is defined as "the area under the blood glucose curve following consumption of 50 g of available carbohydrate from the test food relative to the area under the curve following consumption of 50 g of available carbohydrate from a reference food, either pure glucose or white bread" [213]. By employing glucose as a reference (100), a measured GI less than 55 is regarded as low, a measured GI between 56 and 69 is medium and a measured GI larger than 70 is high [214]. GL is a measure of quantities of saccharides available for providing energy in a food. It is defined as "the product of the amount of available carbohydrate (saccharide) in that serving and the GI of the food" so that it is generally believed that a greater GL of a food results in a higher expected increase in blood glucose and insulin which increases CVD risks [215].

The over-intake of sugars that have high GIs was reported to be associated with an increased risk of myocardial infarction, even when compared with saturated fats [216]. Generally, over-weight or obese body mass caused by the over-intake of saccharides might increase the risk for CVDs, compared to that caused by the over-intake of some fats (including saturated, monosaturated, and polyunsaturated) [217]. A large intake of saccharides (represented as energy percentage (proteins:fats:saccharides), a switch from 15:35:50 to 15:25:60) increased total blood triacylglycerol levels [217,218] and has been suggested to be a higher risk factor of CVDs than blood cholesterol levels [219], since it resulted in insulin resistance [220] [which may cause hyperinsulinemia→dyslipidemia, hypertension, hypofibrinosis, systemic inflammation, and glucose intolerance (→type 2 diabetes) →CVDs]. The saccharide-induced increase in blood triacylglycerol concentrations is elevated with increased body mass index [218]. Controversially, after achieved weight loss, a study indicated that diets improved the lipid profile and decreased CVD risks regardless of which macronutrients they emphasized [221], while another study showed that the benefits of a high-saccharide diet were equal to and only sometimes less than those observed with a high-protein diet [222].

Fructose seems to be the sugar with reported adverse effects on the cardiovascular system. Fructose accounted for 17% of total energy increases fasting total and LDL plasma cholesterols in men, compared to diets nearly devoid of fructose [223], though its adverse effect less than that of sucrose was also reported [224]. Studies in both humans [225] and rats [226] indicated that fructose consumption can increase serum uric acid level, a risk factor for CVDs (see Chapter 8 Overconsumption of Nucleic Acid-increasing Diets for their association with CVDs).

It was recommended that the intake of sugars, mainly including disaccharides (sucrose, lactose, maltose), monosaccharides (glucose, fructose), and mixed sugars (high-fructose corn syrup, honey), should be properly limited (<10% of total energy from free sugars) [227].

Deficiency of Some B Vitamins and CVDs

Folic acid or folate (folacin, also named vitamin B_{11}, VB_{11}), vitamin B_6 (VB_6, or named pyridoxine) and vitamin B_{12} ($VB_{12,}$ or named cyanocobalamin) are essential nutrients. They can not be synthesized in the human body. Therefore, they must be supplied by eating foods or drinking beverages.

Their deficiency should definitely cause the illness of the human body. Therefore, intaking an appropriate amount of foods that are rich in these vitamins should be vital for human health.

Deficiency of Folacin and CVDs

A lack of folacin may result in an estimated 10-25% of deaths from heart diseases and strokes worldwide [228]. Serum folate levels or folate intakes were reported to be inversely associated with cardiovascular endpoints that are independent of serum homocysteine levels [229]. Also, a folate deficiency inhibits the remethylation of homocysteine to methionine, which is a major cause of hyperhomocysteinemia, the established risk factor for CVDs (see Chapter 5 Over Consumption of Homocysteine-increasing Diets). Furthermore, a folate deficiency might have pleiotropic effects on the vascular system, whereas therapeutic responses to various dosages of a folate supplementation could be modified by genetic factors [230]. Therefore, a daily intake of folate higher than Recommended Dietary Allowance (RDA, 400 μg/day for adult men and women, 600 μg/day for pregnant women, and 500 μg/day for lactating women) [183] was suggested to be capable of preventing CVDs [231,232].

Deficiency of Vitamin B_6 and CVDs

A lack of VB_6 may increase homocysteine levels in serum (see Chapter 5 Over Consumption of Homocysteine-increasing Diets) and inflammatory effects that are risk factors for CVDs including those that are not related to the increase in plasma homocysteine levels [233]. The suggested pathway of CVDs associated with a deficiency of VB_6 is summarized in Figure 7.

A plasma VB_6 concentration <20 nmol/L has been previously defined as an insufficient status, whereas <30 nmol/L may be the borderline for the marginal impairment of VB_6 status [183,234].

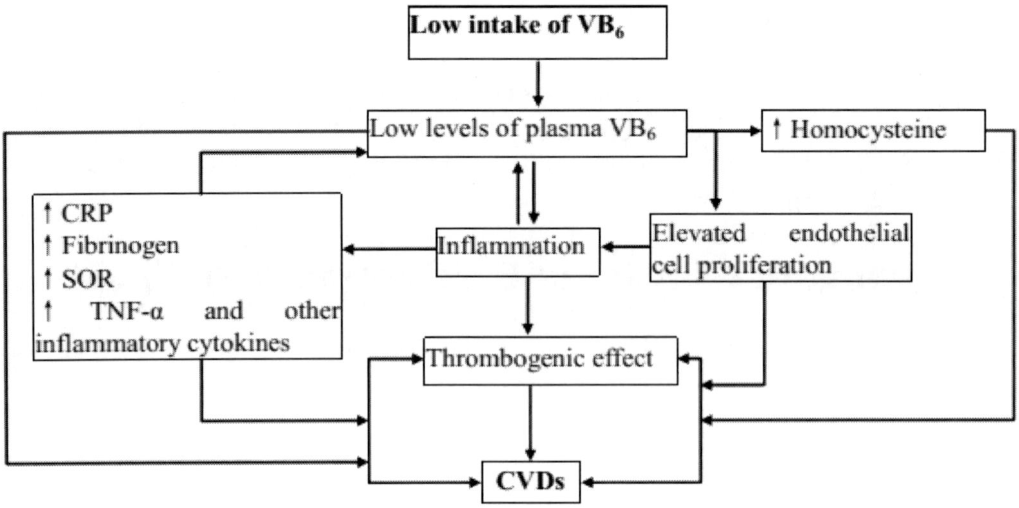

Figure 7. Suggested pathway of CVDs associated with VB_6 deficiency. ↑, increase; SOR, superoxide radicals; TNF-α, tumor necrosis factor-α; CRP, C-reactive protein.

Deficiency of Vitamin B_{12} and CVDs

A lack of VB_{12} may increase homocysteine levels in serum (see Chapter 5 Over Consumption of Homocysteine-increasing Diets) [235,236]. The suggested mechanism is that VB_{12} is a coenzyme for converting 5-methyltetrahydrofolate into hydrofolate involving a remethylation pathway and the metabolism of homocysteine into methionine. It has been reported that 405 μg/mL (300 μmol/L) serum VB_{12} was the cutoff for keeping homocysteine at a healthy level [235].

Although minor conflicting reports can also be found in the literature [237], an overwhelming majority of published papers states that the deficiency of these three B vitamins would increase CVD risks. Therefore, vitamin B therapy may be effective in the prevention of CVDs [238]. On the other hand, it should also be noted that a treatment with B vitamins (doses much higher than the RDA 0.8 mg of folic acid, 0.4 mg of vitamin B_{12}, and 40 mg of vitamin B_6) did not lower the risk of recurrent cardiovascular disease after acute myocardial infarction, which was even suggested to be harmful [239].

Dietary Sources of VB_{11},VB_6 and VB_{12}

The pentaglutamyl conjugate is the predominant form of VB_{11} existing in animal tissues. Its content in the liver can be upto 3 mg/kg while that in muscle tissues is about 30-80 μg/kg. The heptaglutamyl conjugate is the predominant form of VB_{11} existing in leafy green vegetables in which its content is about 200-800 μg/kg. Leafy green vegetables may be the most important sources of VB_{11}. Tetrahydrofolate is the form that acts as a coenzyme. Pteridine in its reduced state is the nucleus of this molecule, connecting with a p-aminobenzoate moiety that carries several glutamate residues (3-7) [240].

VB_6 is found to be present in almost all food resources though its concentration is not high (ca. 100 μg/kg). It is particular rich in wheat germ, egg yolk, meats and other animal tissues, whose concentration is ca. 5 mg/kg. Its content in milk or cheese is ca. 500 μg/kg [240]. The majority of this vitamin may exist as enzyme prosthetic groups in food resources.

It is very unlikely to find VB_{12} in plant food resources. Until now, it is found that this vitamin is only produced by bacteria. Although a trace amount of this vitamin may be found in vegetables, it can almost be sure that it originates from the surface contamination with faeces that are employed as fertilizers. This vitamin is mainly found in animal products, e.g. 200 μg/kg in kidneys, 400 μg/kg in the liver, 10-20 μg/kg in meats, 3 μg/kg in milk and 7 μg/kg in eggs. Most of these animal foods should be very significant sources of this vitamin since 1 μg can meet human's daily requirement. VB_{12} in these food resources should originate from micro-organisms, the consumption of dietary animal products, or synthesized VB_{12} by intestinal micro-organisms with its concentration in the alimentary tract high enough to be absorbed [240].

Deficiency of Vitamin D and CVD

Vitamin D is a compound that is mainly involved in the maintenance and growth of bone tissues. This vitamin is needed to maintain phosphorus and calcium homeostasis. Nevertheless, the function of vitamin D may not be just associated with the maintenance of skeletal health and mineral homeostasis since its receptors are found to be present in other organs and tissues [241].

Vitamin D may not be considered as an essential nutrient and this name may be a misnomer since it can be synthesized in the skin exposing to an ultraviolet B (wavelength being 290 - 315 mm) or sunlight irradiation. The human body can photochemically convert 7-dehydrocholesterol (the precursor) into the most active 1,25-dihy-droxy-vitamin D_3 (1,25-Vit D_3; 1,25-dihydroxycholecalciferol) by a final hydroxylation reaction. However, few sunshine hours during winter, clothing, and modern lifestyle (too much indoor time expended) result in up to 70% vitamin D deficiencies in some population groups [242]. Therefore, food supplements or pharmaceutical applications are now widely practised.

The RDAs for vitamin D are 800 IU/d (15 μg/day) for individuals over 70 years old and 600 IU/d (15 μg/day) for those aged 1 - 70 years, corresponding to a serum 25-hydroxyvitamin D level of ≥50 nmol/L or 20 ng/mL which covers ≥97.5% of the population with the minimal sun exposure [243]. However it should be noted that these RDAs are based on the prevention of bone diseases. They may be different if based on heart health. Recently,

4,000 IU (100 μg) of vitamin D daily has been suggested to be the tolerable upper intake level for the general adult population [244].

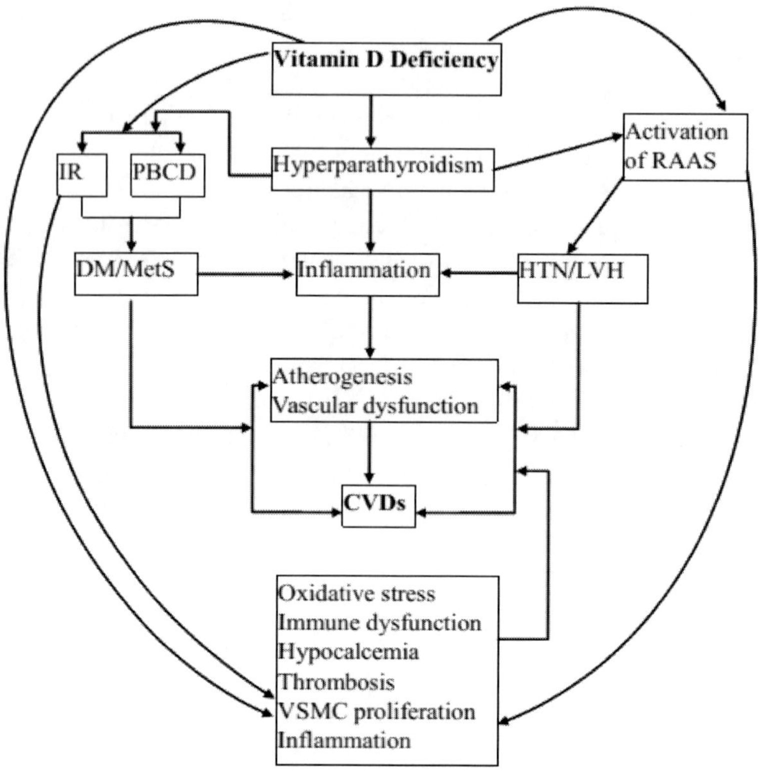

Figure 8. Suggested pathway of CVDs associated with vitamin D deficiency. PBCD, Pancreatic beta cell dysfunction; IR, Insulin resistance DM, Diabetes mellitus; MS, Metabolism syndrome; HTN, Hypertension; LVH, Left ventricular hypertrophy; RAAS, rennin–angiotensin-aldosterone system; VSMC, Vascular smooth muscle cell.

Sources of Vitamin D

Vitamin D_3 (also named cholecalciferol) naturally exists in food resources. It is spectacularly rich in the liver oils of fish, e.g. as high as 15 mg/kg found in mackerel liver oils. Its content in the meat of such fatty fishes as mackerel, herring, and salmon is 50-450 μg/kg. Other food resources that contain vitamin D_3 include milk (1 μg/kg), fatty dairy foods, for example, cream or butter (10-20 μg/kg), egg yolk (60 μg/kg), and all mammalian tissues (<10 μg/kg) [240]. For a food supplementation or pharmaceutical applications, vitamin D_2 is usually used. This form of vitamin D is usually produced by converting a cheap starting material (ergosterol) under an ultraviolet B (290 - 315 mm) irradiation. Plant food resources also contain vitamin D_2 that is also synthesized by converting ergosterol under an ultraviolet B (290 - 315 mm) irradiation.

Deficiency of Vitamin D and CVDs

The deficiency of vitamin D may increase the risk of CVDs, such as ischemic heart disease, myocardial infarction, and early death [245]. It is commonly defined as a plasma level <30 ng/mL of vitamin D [25(OH)D] [246], while the US Institute of Medicine defined plasma levels of <20 ng/mL as being at the risk of vitamin D inadequacy. It was reported that a 78% decrease in type 1 diabetes risks over a 30-year follow-up was achieved by a daily intake of 2,000 IU (50 μg) vitamin D_3 during the first year of life [247]. It was also reported that a daily intake of 1,000 IU (25 μg) vitamin D increased insulin sensitivity or decreased insulin resistance, lowered the levels of fasting insulin with the avoidance of changing the secretion of insulin in a 6-month study including 81 south Asian [248].

Reports on the study and overview of the mechanism or pathway of CVDs associated with the deficiency of vitamin D can be found in the literature [249,250]. The suggested pathway is summarized in Figure 8. In addition, a vitamin D treatment effectively promoted vascular regeneration after a injury in healthy and diabetic subjects [251].

On the other hand, it should also be noted that >50 ng/mL serum vitamin D [25(OH)D] may increase falls, fractures, certain cancers, and even CVD risks [240].

Magnesium Malnutrition and CVDs

Magnesium is essentially required for proper life activities in the body. It is a counter ion for nuclear acids and energy-rich ATP within the cells where it is primarily detected [252]. It acts as a cofactor involving in the reactions of more than 300 enzymes [253,254]. Magnesium critically stabilizes many enzymes, such as those responsible for the generation of ATP [255]. The production of coenzymes, proteins, nucleic acids, and fats, the utilization of glucose, methyl group transfer, muscle contraction and many other processes need ATP and these functions are also affected by the interference of magnesium metabolism [255]. Therefore, it should be noted that the release of neurotransmitters, the function of normal neuroids, the contraction and relaxation of muscles and the metabolism of a ATP are all associated with magnesium. It is also vital to keep in mind that magnesium is associated with the formation of bone, platelet-activated thrombosis, heart rhythm, and the regulation of vascular tone [254,256-259].

Therefore, magnesium is an essential nutrient. They must be supplied by eating foods or drinking beverages.

Dietary Sources of Magnesium

Magnesium widely exists in foods. It can be found in all types of food resources (100-400 mg/kg). Its content can be as high as 0.21% in chlorophylls which is 0.38-1.37 g/kg in selected green leafy vegetables [260], >1.00 g/kg in aquatic animals (by dry matter), most nuts and seeds, most legumes, and most grains or grain products [154].

Magnesium Malnutrition and CVDs

The normal range of blood plasma magnesium concentration in healthy individuals is about 0.7-1.0 mmol/L [261]. The under-intake of magnesium may increase hypertension and other CVD risks [262]. Most reports suggest plasma magnesium levels $\leq$0.61 mmol/L (1.5 mg/dL) being hypomagnesemic [263-265], whereas minor reports considered it $\leq$0.75 mmol/L as being hypomagnesemic [266,267]. Conditions as cirrhosis or cerebrovascular diseases were found to be associated with hypomagnesemia (with a prevalence ranging from 9-65%) [266,268]. The mechanism of association of hypomagnesemia with CVDs may involve: over-producing coagulation factors (protrombin, thrombin, V, VII, IX), inducing cells unable to retain K differences between the intra- and extra-cellular space and ensuing intracellular K depletion because of the dependence of Na/K pump on Mg, promoting lesions in arteries, and causing endothelial dysfunction (increased E-selectin) and inflammation (increased CRP, the biomarker).

Conversely, hypermagnesium may also have adverse cardiac effects such as atrial fibrillation and bradycardia [268]. Bradycardia was observed at doses of serum magnesium levels being 2.1 – 2.4 mmol/L [269,270].

Therefore, the cutting point of the proper hypermagnesium level may be in the range of >1.0 in plasma and <2.1 mmol/L in serum.

References

[1] WHO., Obesity: preventing and managing the global epidemic. Report of a WHO consultation. World Health Organ Tech Rep Ser 894(i–xii); 2000; pp.1-253.

[2] Kuczmarski, R.J., Ogden, C.L., Grummer-Strawn, L.M., Flegal, K.M., Guo, S.S., Wei, R., Mei, Z., Curtin, L.R., Roche, A.F., Johnson, C.L., (2000). CDC growth charts: United States. *Adv. Data.* 314,1-27.

[3] Janssen, I., Katzmarzyk, P.T., Ross, R., (2002). Body mass index, waist circumference, and health risk: evidence in support of current National Institutes of Health guidelines. *Arch. Intern. Med.* 162(18), 2074-9.

[4] Constantine, T., Hainer, V., Basdevant, A., Finer, N., Fried, M. Mathus-Vliegen, E., Micic, D., Maislos, M., Roman, G. Schutz, Y. Toplak, H., Zahorska-Markiewicz, B., (2008). Management of Obesity in Adults: European Clinical Practice Guidelines. *Obes. Facts* 1(2), 106-16.

[5] Okorodudu, D.O., Jumean, M.F., Montori, V.M., Romero-Corral, A., Somers, V.K., Erwin, P.J., Lopez-Jimenez, F., (2010). Diagnostic performance of body mass index to identify obesity as defined by body adiposity: a systematic review and meta-analysis. *Internat. J. Obes.* 34, 791-799.

[6] Yusuf, S., Hawken, S., Ounpuu, S., Dans, T., Avezum, A., Lanas, F., McQueen, M., Budaj, A., Pais, P., Varigos, J., Lisheng, L., (2004). Effect of potentially modifiable risk factors associated with myocardial infarction in 52 countries (the INTERHEART study): Case-control study. *Lancet.* 364(9438), 937-52.

[7] Bergman, R.N., Stefanovski, D., Buchanan, T.A., Sumner, A.E., Reynolds, J.C., Sebring, N.G., Anny H. Xiang, A.H., Richard M. Watanabe, R.M., (2011). A Better Index of Body adiposity. *Obesity* 19, 1083-1089.

[8] Lemacks, J.L., Liu, P.Y., Shin, H., Ralston, P.A., Ilich, J.Z., (2012). Validation of body adiposity index as a measure of obesity in overweight and obese postmenopausal white women and its comparison with body mass index. *Menopause* 19(11), 1277-9.

[9] Gibson, C.D., Atalayer, D., Flancbaum, L., Geliebter, A., (2012). Body adiposity index (BAI) correlates with BMI and body fat pre- and post-bariatric surgery but is not an adequate substitute for BMI in severely obese women. *Int. J. Body Compos. Res.* 10(1), 9-14.

[10] Acheson, K.J., Schulz, Y., Bessard, T., Flatt, J.P., Jéquier, E., (1987). Carbohydrate metabolism and de novo lipogenesis in human obesity. *Am. J. Clin. Nutr.* 45, 78-85.

[11] Acheson, K.J., Schutz, Y., Bessard, T., Flatt, J.P., Jéquier, E., (1998). Glycogen storage capacity and de novo lipogenesis during massive carbohydrate overfeeding in men. *Am. J. Clin. Nutri.* 48, 240-247.

[12] Klok, M.D., Jakobsdottir, S., Drent, M.L., (2007). The role of leptin and ghrelin in the regulation of food intake and body weight in humans: a review. *Obes. Rev.* 8, 21-34.

[13] Byatt, J.C., Staten, N.R., Salsgiver, W.J., Kostelc, J.G., Collier, R.J., (1993). Stimulation of food intake and weight gain in mature female rats by bovine prolactin and bovine growth hormone. *Am. J. Physiol.* 264, E986–E992.

[14] Roberts, T.J., Azain, M.J., (1995). Effect of somatotropin on rate and composition of gain and feed intake in young, pituitary intact female rats. *Growth Develop. Aging* 59, 3–13.

[15] Vasilatos-Younken, R., Wang, X.H., Zhou, Y., Day, J.R., Mcmutry, J.P., Rosebrough, R.W., Decuypere, E., Buys, N., Darras, V.M., Beard, J.L., Tomas, F., (1999). New insights into the mechanism and actions of growth hormone (GH) in poultry. *Domest. Anim. Endocrinol.* 17, 181-190.

[16] Malmlöf, K., Din, N., Johansen, T., Pedersen, S.B., (2002). Growth hormone affects both adiposity and voluntary food intake in old and obese female rats. *Europ. J. Endocrinol.* 146, 121-128.

[17] Wren, A.M., Seal, L.J., Cohen, M.A., Brynes, A.E., Frost, G.S., Murphy, K.G., Dhillo, W.S., Ghatei, M.A., Bloom, S.R., (2001). Ghrelin enhances appetite and increases food intake in humans. *J. Clin. Endocrinol. Metab.* 86, 5992-5995.

[18] Tassone, F., Broglio, F., Destefanis, S., Rovere, S., Benso, A., Gottero, C., Prodam, F., Rossetto, R., Gauna, C., van der Lely, A.J., Ghigo, E., Maccario, M., (2003). Neuroendocrine and metabolic effects of acute ghrelin administration in human obesity. *J. Clin. Endocrinol. Metab.* 88, 5478-5483.

[19] Schmid, D.A., Held, K., Ising, M., Uhr, M., Weikel, J.C., Steiger, A., (2005). Ghrelin stimulates appetite, imagination of food, GH, ACTH, and cortisol, but does not affect leptin in normal controls. *Neuropsychopharmacol.* 30, 1187-1192.

[20] Hukshorn, C.J., Saris, W.H., Westerterp-Plantenga, M.S., Farid, A.R., Smith, F.J., Campfield, L.A., (2000). Weekly subcutaneous pegylated recombinant native human leptin (PEG-OB) administration in obese men. *J. Clin. Endocrinol. Metab.* 85, 4003-4009.

[21] Caro, J.F., Kolaczynski, J.W., Nyce, M.R., Ohannesian, J.P., Opentanova, I., Goldman, W.H., Lynn, R.B., Zhang, P.L., Sinha, M.K., Considine, R.V., (1996). Decreased

cerebrospinal-fluid/serum leptin ratio in obesity: a possible mechanism for leptin resistance. *Lancet.* 348, 159-161.

[22] Glavas, M.M., Kirigiti, M.A., Xiao, X.Q., Enriori, P.J., Fisher, S.K., Evans, A.E., Grayson, B.E., Cowley, M.A., Smith, M.S., Grove, K.L., (2010). Early Overnutrition Results in Early-Onset Arcuate Leptin Resistance and Increased Sensitivity to High-Fat Diet. *Endocrinol.* 151, 1598-1610.

[23] Fuhrman, J., Sarter, B., Glaser, D., Acocella, S., (2010). Changing perceptions of hunger on a high nutrient density diet. *Nutr. J.* 29, 51-63.

[24] Chiu, K.C., Chu, A., Go, V.L., Saad, M.F., (2004). Hypovitaminosis D is associated with insulin resistance and cell dysfunction. *Am. J. Clin. Nutr.* 79, 820-5.

[25] Kleefstra, N., Bilo, H.J., Bakker, S.J., Houweling, S.T., (2004). Chromium and insulin resistance (Article in Dutch). *Ned. Tijdschr. Geneeskd.* 148(5), 217-20.

[26] Nadler, J.L., Buchanan, T., Natarajan, R., Antonipillai, I., Bergman, R., Rude, R., (1993). Magnesium deficiency produces insulin resistance and increased thromboxane synthesis. *Hypertens.* 21(6 Pt 2), 1024-9.

[27] Fargion, S., Dongiovanni, P., Guzzo, A., Colombo, S., Valenti, L., Fracanzani, A.L., (2005). Iron and insulin resistance. *Aliment. Pharmacol. Ther.* 22(Suppl 2), 61-3.

[28] Taneja, S.K., Mandal, R., Chechi, A., (2012). Attenuation of Zn-induced hyperleptinemia/leptin resistance in Wistar rat after feeding modified poultry egg. *Nutr. Metab.* 9, 85-93.

[29] Steinbrenner, H., Speckmann, B., Pinto, A., Sies, H., (2011). High selenium intake and increased diabetes risk: experimental evidence for interplay between selenium and carbohydrate metabolism. *J. Clin. Biochem. Nutr.* 48(1), 40-45.

[30] Ristow, M., Zarse, K., Oberbach, A., Klöting, N., Birringer, M., Kiehntopf, M., Stumvoll, M., Kahn, C.R., Blüher, M., (2009). Antioxidants prevent healthpromoting effects of physical exercise in humans. *Proc. Natl. Acad. Sci. USA* 106, 8665-8670.

[31] Roden, M., Price, T.B., Perseghin, G., Petersen, K.F., Rothman, D.L., Cline, G.W., Shulman, G.I., (1996). Mechanism of free fatty-acid induced insulin resistance in humans. *J. Clin. Invest.* 97, 2859-2865.

[32] Kawanaka, K., Han, D.H., Gao, J., Nolte, L.A., Holloszy, J.O., (2001). Development of Glucose-induced Insulin Resistance in Muscle Requires Protein Synthesis. *J. Biol. Chem.* 276, 20101-20107.

[33] Krebs, M., Krssak, M., Bernroider, E., Anderwald, C., Brehm, A., Meyerspeer, M., Nowotny, P., Erich Roth, E., Waldhäusl, W., Roden, M., (2002). Mechanism of Amino Acid-Induced Skeletal Muscle Insulin Resistance in Humans. *Diabetes* 51(3), 599-605.

[34] White, C.L., Whittington, A., Barnes, M.J., Wang, Z., Bray, G.A., Morrison, C.D., (2009). HF diets increase hypothalamic PTP1B and induce leptin resistance through both leptin-dependent and -independent mechanisms. *Am. J. Physiol. Endocrinol. Metab.* 296, E291–E299.

[35] O'Dea, K., (1991). Westernization and non-insulin-dependent diabetes in Australian Aborigines. *Ethn. Dis.* 1, 171–87.

[36] Steinberg, G.R., Dyck, D.J., (2000). Development of leptin resistance in rat soleus muscle in response to high-fat diets. *Am. J. Physiol. Endocrinol. Metab.* 279, E1374–E1382.

[37] Banks, W.A., Coon, A.B., Robinson, S.M., Moinuddin, A., Shultz, J.M., Nakaoke, R., Morley, J.E., (2004). Triglycerides Induce Leptin Resistance at the Blood-Brain Barrier. *Diabetes* 53, 1253–1260.

[38] Shapiro, A., Mu, W., Roncal, C., Cheng, K.Y., Johnson, R.J., Scarpace, P.J., (2008). Fructose-Induced Leptin Resistance Exacerbates Weight Gain in Response to Subsequent High Fat Feeding. *Am. J. Physiol. Regul. Integr. Comp. Physiol.* 295(5), R1370–R1375.

[39] Basciano, H., Federico, L., Adeli, K., (2005). Fructose, insulin resistance, and metabolic dyslipidemia. *Nutr. Metab.* 2, 5-18.

[40] Byrens, S.E., Miller, J.C.B., Denver, G.S., (1995). Amylopectin Starch Promotes the Development of Insulin Resistance in Rats. *J. Nutr.* 125, 1430-1437.

[41] Pereira, M.A., Jacobs, D.R., Van Horn, L., Slattery, M.L., Kartashov, A.I., Ludwig, D.S., (2002). Dairy consumption, obesity, and the insulin resistance syndrome in young adults: the CARDIA Study. *JAMA*. 287, 2081-2089.

[42] Te Morenga, L.A., Levers, M.T., Williams, S.M., Brown, R.C., Mann, J., (2011). Comparison of high protein and high fiber weight-loss diets in women with risk factors for the metabolic syndrome: a randomized trial. *Nutr. J.* 10, 40-48.

[43] Hoppe, C., Molgaard, C., Vaag, A., Barkholt, V., Michaelsen, K.F., (2005). High intakes of milk, but not meat, increase s-insulin and insulin resistance in 8-year-old boys. *Eur. J. Clin. Nutr.* 59, 393– 8.

[44] Jönsson, T., Olsson, S., Ahrén, B., Bøg-Hansen, T.C., Dole, A., Lindeberg, S., (2005). Agrarian diet and diseases of affluence- Do evolutionary novel dietary lectins cause leptin resistance? *BMC Endocr. Disord.* 5, 10. doi:10.1186/1472-6823-5-10.

[45] Fraze, E., Chlou, M., Chen, Y., Reaven, G.M., (1987). Age related changes in postprandial plasma glucose, insulin, and FFA concentrations in non-diabetic individuals. *J. Am. Geriatr. Soc.* 35, 224-228.

[46] Gabriely, I., Ma, X.H., Yang, X.M., Rossetti, L., Barzilai, N., (2002). Leptin Resistance During Aging Is Independent of Fat Mass. *Diabetes* 51, 1016 –1021.

[47] Van Cauter, E., (2011). Sleep disturbances and insulin resistance. *Diabet. Med.* 28(12), 1455-62.

[48] Schmid, S.M., Hallschmid, M., Jauch-Chara, K., Born, J., Schultes, B., (2008). A single night of sleep deprivation increases ghrelin levels and feelings of hunger in normal-weight healthy men. *J. Sleep Res.* 17, 331-334.

[49] Lyytikäinen, P., Rahkonen, O., Lahelma, E., Lallukka, T., (2011). Association of sleep duration with weight and weight gain: a prospective follow-up study. *J. Sleep Res.* 20, 98-302.

[50] Rajagopalan, S., Brook, R.D., (2012). Air pollution and type 2 diabetes: mechanistic insights. *Diabetes* 61, 3037-3045.

[51] Thiering, E., Cyrys, J., Kratzsch, J., Meisinger, C., Hoffmann, B., Berdel, D., von Berg, A., Koletzko, S., Bauer, C.P., Heinrich, J., (2013). Long-term exposure to traffic-related air pollution and insulin resistance in children: results from the GINIplus and LISAplus birth cohorts. *Diabetologia* 56, 1696–1704.

[52] Elmquist, J.K., Elias, C.F., Saper, C.B., (1999). From lesions to leptin: hypothalamic control of food intake and body weight. *Neuron.* 22, 221–232.

[53] Suga, A., Hirano, T., Kageyama, H., Kashiba, M., Oka, J., Osaka, T., Namba, Y., Tsuji, M., Miura, M., Adachi, M., Inoue, S., (1999). Rapid increase in circulating leptin in

ventromedial hypothalamus-lesioned rats: role of hyperinsulinemia and implication for upregulation mechanism. *Diabetes* 48(10), 2034-8.
[54] Stricker, E.M., Rowland, N., (1978). Hepatic versus cerebral origin of stimulus for feeding induced by 2-deoxy-d-glucose in rats. *J. Comp. Physiol. Psychol.* 92, 126 –132.
[55] Duggan, J.P., Booth, D.A., (1986). Obesity, overeating, and rapid gastric emptying in rats with ventromedial hypothalamic lesions. *Science* 231, 609–611.
[56] Rohner-Jeanrenaud, F., Jeanrenaud, B., (1980). Consequences of Ventromedial Hypothalamic Lesions upon Insulin and Glucagon Secretion by Subsequently Isolated Perfused Pancreases in the Rat. *J. Clin. Invest.* 65, 902-910.
[57] Olney, J.W., (1969). Brain lesions, obesity, and other disturbances in mice treated with monosodium glutamate. *Science* 164, 719–721.
[58] Cassidy, S.B., (1997). Prader-Willi syndrome. *J. Med. Genet.* 34(11), 917–23.
[59] Beales, P., Elcioglu, N., Woolf, A., Parker, D., Flinter, F., (1999) New criteria for improved diagnosis of Bardet–Biedl syndrome: results of a population survey. *J. Med. Genet.* 36(6), 437–46.
[60] Feuillan, P.P., Ng, D., Han, J.C., Sapp, J.C., Wetsch, K., Spaulding, E., Zheng, Y.C., Caruso, R.C., Brooks, B.P., Johnston, J.J., Yanovski, J.A., Biesecker, L.G., (2011). Patients with Bardet-Biedl Syndrome Have Hyperleptinemia Suggestive of Leptin Resistance. *J. Clin. Endocrinol. Metab.* 96(3), E528–E535.
[61] Kolehmainen, J., Black, G.C., Saarinen, A., Chandler, K., Clayton-Smith, J., Träskelin, A.L., Perveen, R., Kivitie-Kallio, S., Norio, R., Warburg, M., Fryns, J.P., de la Chapelle, A., Lehesjoki, A.E., (2003). Cohen syndrome is caused by mutations in a novel gene, COH1, encoding a transmembrane protein with a presumed role in vesicle-mediated sorting and intracellular protein transport. *Am. J. Hum. Genet.* 72(6), 1359–69.
[62] Massa, G., Dooms, L., Vanderschueren-Lodeweyckx, M.., (1991). Growth hormone deficiency in a girl with the Cohen syndrome. *J. Med. Genet.* 28, 48-50.
[63] Adams, M., Smith, U.M., Logan, C.V., Johnson, C.A., (2008). Recent advances in the molecular pathology, cell biology and genetics of ciliopathies. *J. Med. Genet. (BMJ)* 45(5), 257–267.
[64] Morgan, T., (2007). Turner Syndrome: diagnosis and management. *Am. Fam. Physician.* 76, 405-410.
[65] Moretti-Ferreira, D., Koiffmann, C.P., Listik, M., Setian, N., Wajntal, A., (1993). Macrosomia, obesity, macrocephaly and ocular abnormalities (MOMO syndrome) in two unrelated patients: delineation of a newly recognized overgrowth syndrome. *Am. J. Med. Genet.* 46(5), 555–8.
[66] Schumann, R.R., Leong, S.R., Flaggs, G.W., Gray, P.W., Wright, S.D., Mathison, J.C., Tobias, P.S., Ulevitch, R.J., (1990). Structure and function of lipopolysaccharide binding protein. *Science* 249, 1429–1431.
[67] Backhed, F., Ding, H., Wang, T., Hooper, L.V., Koh, G.Y.Y., Nagy, A., Semenkovich, C.F., Gordon, J.I., (2004). The gut microbiota as an environmental factor that regulates fat storage. *Proc. Natl. Acad. Sci. USA* 101, 15718–15723.
[68] Cani, P.D., Amar, J., Iglesias, M.A., Poggi, M., Knauf, C., Bastelica, D., Neyrinck, A.M., Fava, F., Tuohy, K.M., Chabo, C., Waget, A., Delmée, E., Cousin, B., Sulpice, T., Chamontin, B., Ferrières, J., Tanti, J.F., Gibson, G.R., Casteilla, L., Delzenne, N.M.,

Alessi, M.C., Burcelin, R., (2007). Metabolic endotoxemia initiates obesity and insulin resistance. *Diabetes* 56, 1761–1772.

[69] Castinetti, F., Morange, I., Conte-Devolx, B., Brue, T., (2012). Cushing's disease. *Orphanet. J. Rare Dis.* 7, 41-49.

[70] McTiernan, A., (2005). Obesity and cancer: the risks, science, and potential management strategies. *Oncol.* 19, 871–81.

[71] Otake, S., Takeda, H., Suzuki, Y., Fukui, T., Watanabe, S., Ishihama, K., Saito, T., Togashi, H., Nakamura, T., Matsuzawa, Y., Kawata, S., (2005). Association of visceral fat accumulation and plasma adiponectin with colorectal adenoma: evidence for participation of insulin resistance. *Clin. Cancer Res.* 11, 3642–6.

[72] Stoll, B.A., (1999). Western nutrition and the insulin resistance syndrome: a link to breast cancer. *Eur. J. Clin. Nutr.* 53, 83–7.

[73] Martin, R.L., Perez, E., He, Y.J., Dawson, R., Millard, W.J., (2000). Leptin resistance is associated with hypothalamic leptin receptor mRNA and protein downregulation. *Metab.* 49, 1479 –1484.

[74] Fukuda, M., Williams, K.W., Gautron, L., Elmquist, J.K., (2011). Induction of Leptin Resistance by Activation of cAMP-Epac Signaling. *Cell Metab.* 13, 331–339.

[75] Scarpace, P.J., Matheny, M., Zhang, Y., Shek, E.W., Prima, V., Zolotukhin, S., Tümer, N., (2002). Leptin-Induced Leptin Resistance Reveals Separate Roles for the Anorexic and Thermogenic Responses in Weight Maintenance. *Endocrinol.* 143(8), 3026-3035.

[76] Maier, V.H., Gould, G.W., (2000). Long-term insulin treatment of 3T3-L1 adipocytes results in mis-targeting of GLUT4: implications for insulin-stimulated glucose transport. *Diabetologia* 43(10), 1273-81.

[77] Harder, T., Plagemann, A., Rohde, W., Dorner, G., (1998). Syndrome X-like alterations in adult female rats due to neonatal insulin treatment. *Metab.* 47, 855-62.

[78] Harder, T., Rake, A., Rohde, W., Doerner, G., Plagemann, A., (1999). Overweight and increased diabetes susceptibility in neonatally insulin-treated adult rats. *Endocr. Regul.* 33, 25-31.

[79] Masharani, U.B., Maddux, B.A., Li, X., Sakkas, G.K., Mulligan, K., Schambelan, M., Goldfine, I.D., Youngren, J.F., (2011). Insulin Resistance in Non-Obese Subjects Is Associated with Activation of the JNK Pathway and Impaired Insulin Signaling in Skeletal Muscle. *PLoS ONE* 6(5), e19878.

[80] Smith, T.R., Elmendorf, J.S., David, T.S., Turinsky, J., (1997). Growth hormone-induced insulin resistance: role of the insulin receptor, IRS-1, GLUT-1, and GLUT-4. *Am. J. Physiol.* 272, E1071–E1079.

[81] Thirone, A.C., Carvalho, C.R., Brenelli, S.L., Velloso, L.A., Saad, M.J., (1997). Effect of chronic growth hormone treatment on insulin signal transduction in rat tissues. *Mol. Cell Endocrinol.* 130, 33– 42.

[82] Solano, J.M., Jacobson, L., (1999). Glucocorticoids reverse leptin effects on food intake and body fat in mice without increasing NPY mRNA. *Am. J. Physiol. Endocrinol. Metab.* 277, E708-E716.

[83] Di, S., Malcher-Lopex, R., Halmos, K.C., Tasker, J.G., (2003). Nongenomic glucocorticoid inhibition via endocannabinoid release in the hypothalamus: a fast feedback mechanism. *J. Neurosci.* 23, 4850–4857.

[84] Widmaier, E.P., Dallman, M.F., (1984). The effects of corticotropin-releasing factor on adrenocorticotropin secretion from perifused pituitaries in vitro: rapid inhibition by glucocorticoids. *Endocrinol.* 115, 2368-2374.

[85] Augustine, R.A., Grattan, D.R., (2008). Induction of Central Leptin Resistance in Hyperphagic Pseudopregnant Rats by Chronic Prolactin Infusion. *Endocrinol.* 149(3), 1049-1055

[86] Deibert, D.C., DeFronzo, R.A., (1980). Epinephrine-induced insulin resistance in man. *J. Clin. Invest.* 65, 717-721.

[87] Bailey, C.J., Turner, S.L., (2004). Glucosamine-induced insulin resistance in L6 muscle cells. *Diabetes Obes. Metab.* 6(4), 293-8.

[88] Keijzers, G.B., De Galan, B.E., Tack, C.J., Smits, P., (2002). Caffeine Can Decrease Insulin Sensitivity in Humans. *Diabetes Care* 25, 364-369.

[89] Biaggioni, I., Davis, S., (2002). Caffeine: A Cause of Insulin Resistance? *Diabetes Care* 25(2), 399-400.

[90] Blagosklonny, M.V., (2012). Once again on rapamycin-induced insulin resistance and longevity: despite of or to. *Aging* 4(5), 350-358.

[91] Penhos, J.C., Lazarus, N.R., Yamaguchi, N., Gutman, R.A., Recant, L., (1972). Insulin-resistant hyperglycemia produced by aminophylline. *Isr. J. Med. Sci.* 8, 917-918.

[92] Holscher, C., van Aalten, L., Sutherland, C., (2008). Anaesthesia generates neuronal insulin resistance by inducing hypothermia. *BMC Neurosci.* 9, 100.

[93] Lund, L.H., Freda, P., Williams, J.J., LaManca, J.J., LeJemtel, T.H., Mancini, D.M., (2010). Leptin resistance after heart transplantation. *Eur. J. Heart Fail.* 12, 516-520.

[94] Williams, J.J., Lund, L.H. LaManca, J., Kunavarapu, C., Cohen, D.J., Heshka, S., Heymsfield, S.B., Mancini, D.M., (2006). Excessive weight gain in cardiac transplant recipients. *J. Heart Lung Transplant.* 25, 36-41.

[95] Baessler, A., Hasinoff, M.J., Fischer, M., Reinhard, W., Sonnenberg, G.E., Olivier, M., Erdmann, J., Schunkert, H., Doering, A., Jacob, H.J., Comuzzie, A.G., Kissebah, A.H., Kwitek, A.E., (2005). Genetic linkage and association of the growth hormone secretagogue receptor (ghrelin receptor) gene in human obesity. *Diabetes* 54, 259-267.

[96] Silventoinen, K., Kaprio, J., (2009). Genetics of tracking of body mass index from birth to late middle age: evidence from twin and family studies. *Obes. Facts* 2, 196-202.

[97] Volkow, N.D., Wang, G.J., Baler, R.D., (2011). Reward, dopamine and the control of food intake: implications for obesity. *Trends Cogn. Sci.* 15(1), 37-46.

[98] Bell, C.G., Walley, A.J., Froguel, P., (2005). THE GENETICS OF HUMAN OBESITY. *Nat. Rev. Gen.* 6, 221-234.

[99] Volkow, N.D., Wang, G.J., Tomasi, D., Baler, R.D., (2013). Obesity and addiction: neurobiological overlaps. *Obes. Rev.* 14, 2-18.

[100] Orosco, M., Rouch, C., Nicolaidis, S., (1996). Rostromedial hypothalamic monoamine changes in response to intravenous infusions of insulin and glucose in freely feeding obese Zucker rats: a microdialysis study. *Appetite* 26, 1-20

[101] Geiger, B.M., Haburcak, M., Avena, N.M., Moeyer, M.C., Hoebel, B.G., Photos, E.N., (2009). Deficits of mesolimbic dopamine neurotransmission in rat dietary obesity. *Neurosci.* 159(4), 1193–1199.

[102] Arias-Carrión, O., Pöppel, E., (2007). Dopamine, learning and reward-seeking behavior. *Act Neurobiol. Exp.* 67(4), 481-488.

[103] Berridge, K., (2009). 'Liking' and 'wanting' food rewards: brain substrates and roles in eating disorders. *Physiol. Behav.* 97, 537-550.

[104] de Oliveira, E., Moura, E.G., Santos-Silva, A.P., Pinheiro, C.P., Lima, N.S., Nogueira-Neto, J.F., Nunes-Freitas, A.L., Abreu-Villaça, Y., Passos, M.C.F., Lisboa, P.C., (2010). Neonatal nicotine exposure causes insulin and leptin resistance and inhibits hypothalamic leptin signaling in adult rat offspring. *J. Endocrinol.* 206, 55-63.

[105] Davis, C.A., Levitan, R.D., Reid, C., Carter, J.C., Kaplan, A.S., Patte, K.A., King, N., Curtis, C., Kennedy, J.L., (2009). Dopamine for 'wanting' and opioids for 'liking': a comparison of obese adults with and without binge eating. *Obesity (Silver Spring)* 17, 1220-1225.

[106] Van Gaal, L.F., Vansant, G.A., Leeuw, I.H.D., (1992). Factors determining energy expenditure during very-low-calorie diets. *Am. J. Clin. Nutr.* 56, 224S-9S.

[107] Ebbeling, C.B., Swain, J.F., Feldman, H.A., Wong, W.W., Hachey, D.L., Garcia-Lago, E., Ludwig, D.S., (2012). Effects of Dietary Composition on Energy Expenditure During Weight-Loss Maintenance. *JAMA.* 307(24), 2627-2634.

[108] Guntur, A.R., Rosen, C.J., (2012). Bone as an Endocrine Organ. *Endocr. Pract.* 18(5), 758-762.

[109] Yamashita, Y., Kaya, M., Koyama, K., Tsujita, J., Hori, S., (2005). Decreased energy expenditure during prolonged sub-maximal exercise in a warm environment. *Eur. J. Sport Sci.* 5(4), 153-158.

[110] Takahashi, H., Nishikawa, T., Mizutani, T., Handa, F., (1997). Oral clonidine premedication decreases energy expenditure in human volunteers. *Can. J. Anaesth.* 44(3), 268-272.

[111] Williams, R., Olivi, S., Li, C.S., Storm, M., Cremer, L., Mackert, P., Wang, W., (2004). Oral glutamine supplementation decreases resting energy expenditure in children and adolescents with sickle cell anemia. *J. Pediatr. Hematol. Oncol.* 26(10), 619-25.

[112] Bekx, M.T., Carrel, A.L., Shriver, T.C., Li, Z., Allen, D.B., (2003). Decreased energy expenditure is caused by abnormal body composition in infants with Prader-Willi Syndrome. *J. Pediatr.* 143(3), 372-6.

[113] Danforth, E., Burger, A.G., (1984). The role of thyroid hormones in the control of energy expenditure. *Clin. Endocrin. Metab.* 13, 581–595.

[114] Santosa, S., Khosla, S., McCready, L.K., Jensen, M.D., (2010). Effects of Estrogen and Testosterone on Resting Energy Expenditure in Older Men. *Obesity* 18(12), 2392–2394.

[115] Daenzer, M., Ortmann, S., Klaus, S., Metges, C.C., (2002). Prenatal High Protein Exposure Decreases Energy Expenditure and Increases Adiposity in Young Rats. *J. Nutr.* 132(2), 142-144.

[116] Glick, M., Segal-Lieberman, G., Cohen, R., Kronfeld-Schor, N., (2009). Chronic MCH infusion causes a decrease in energy expenditure and body temperature, and an increase in serum IGF-1 levels in mice. *Endocrine* 36(3), 479-485.

[117] Benedict, C., Hallschmid, M., Lassen, A., Mahnke, C., Schultes, B., Schiöth, H.B., Born, J., Lange, T., (2011). Acute sleep deprivation reduces energy expenditure in healthy men. *Am. J. Clin. Nutr.* 93(6), 1229-1236.

[118] Vaughan, L., Zurlo, F., Ravussin, E., (1991). Aging and energy expenditure. *Am. J. Clin. Nutr.* 53, 821-825.

[119] Day, D.S., Gozansky, W.S., Van Pelt, R.E., Schwartz, R.S., Kohrt, W.M., (2005). Sex Hormone Suppression Reduces Resting Energy Expenditure and β-Adrenergic Support of Resting Energy Expenditure. *J. Clin. Endocrinol. Metab.* 90(6), 3312-3317.

[120] Klausen, B., Toubro, S., Astrup, A., (1997). Age and sex effects on energy expenditure. *Am. J. Clin. Nutr.* 65(4), 895-907.

[121] Westerterp, K.R., (2004). Diet induced thermogenesis. *Nutri. Metab.* 1, 1-5.

[122] Meijer, G.A.L., Janssen, G.M.E., Westerterp, K.R., Verhoeven, F., Saris, W.H.M., ten Hoor, F., (1991). The effect of a 5-month endurance-training programme on physical acitivity: evidence for a sex-difference in the metabolic response to excise. *Eur. J. Appl. Physiol.* 62, 11-17.

[123] Arble, D.M., Bass, J., Laposky, A.D., Vitaterna, M.H., Turek, F.W., (2009). Circadian Timing of Food Intake Contributes to Weight Gain. *Obesity* 17, 2100-2102.

[124] Damiola, F., Le Minh, N., Preitner, N., Kornmann, B., Fleury-Olela, F., Schibler, U., (2000). Restricted feeding uncouples circadian oscillators in peripheral tissues from the central pacemaker in the suprachiasmatic nucleus. *Genes Dev.* 14, 2950-2961.

[125] Cleator, J., Abbott, J., Judd, P., Sutton, C., Wilding, J.P.H., (2012). Night eating syndrome: implications for severe obesity. *Nutr. Diabetes* 2, e44. doi:10.1038/nutd.2012.16.

[126] Vik, T., Jacobsen, G., Vatten, L., Bakketeig, L.S., (1996). Pre- and post-natal growth in children of women who smoked in pregnancy. *Early Hum. Develop.* 19, 245-255.

[127] Blake, K.V., Gurrin, L.C., Evans, S.F., Beilin, L.J., Landau, L.I., Stanley, F.J., Newnham, J.P., (2000). Maternal cigarette smoking during pregnancy, low birth weight and subsequent blood pressure in early childhood. *Early Hum. Develop.* 57, 137-147.

[128] Von Kries, R., Toschke, A.M., Koletzko, B., Slikker, W., (2002). Maternal smoking during pregnancy and childhood obesity. *Am. J. Epidemiol.* 15, 6954-961.

[129] Chen, W.J., Kelly, R.B., (2005). Effect of prenatal or perinatal nicotine exposure on neonatal thyroid status and offspring growth in rats. *Life Sci.* 76, 1249-1258.

[130] Gao, Y.J., Holloway, A.C., Zeng, Z.H., Lim, G.E., Petrik, J.J., Foster, W.G., Lee, R.M., (2005). Prenatal exposure to nicotine causes postnatal obesity and altered perivascular adipose tissue function. *Obes. Res.* 3, 687-692.

[131] Goldani, M.Z., Haeffner, L.S.B., Agranonik, M., Barbieri, M.A., Bettiol, H., Silva, A.A.M., (2007). Do early life factors influence body mass index in adolescents? *Braz. J. Med. Biol. Res.* 40, 1231-1236.

[132] Guiraudou, M., Varlet-Marie, E., Raynaud de Mauverger, E., Brun, J.F., (2013). Obesity-related increase in whole blood viscosity includes different profiles according to fat localization. *Clin. Hemorheol. Microcirc.* 55(1), 63-73.

[133] Kotsis, V., Stabouli, S., Papakatsika, S., Rizos, Z., Parati, G., (2010). Mechanisms of obesity-induced hypertension. *Hypertens. Res.* 33, 386–393.

[134] Nelson, R., (2013). Hyperlipidemia as a Risk Factor for Cardiovascular Disease. *Prim. Care.* 40(1), 195–211.

[135] Lowe, G.D.O., Blood rheology and vascular disease. Haemostasis and Thrombosis (ed. by A.L. Bloom et al.), 3rd edn. Churchill Livingstone, Edinburgh; 1994; pp.1169-1188.

[136] de Simone, G., Devereux, R.B., Chien, S., Alderman, M.H., Atlas, S.A., Laragh, J.H., (1990). Relation of Blood Viscosit to Demographic and Physiologic Variables and to Cardiovascular Risk Factors in Apparently Normal Adults. *Circulation* 81, 107-117.

[137] Késmárky G, Kenyeres P, Rábai M, Tóth K., (2008). Plasma viscosity: a forgotten variable. *Clin Hemorheol. Microcirc.* 39(1-4), 243–6.

[138] Koenig, W., Sund, M., Filipiak, B., Döring, A., Löwel, H., Ernst, E., (1998). Plasma Viscosity and the Risk of Coronary Heart Disease: Results From the MONICA-Augsburg Cohort Study, 1984 to 1992. *Arterioscler. Thromb. Vasc. Biol.* 18, 768-772.

[139] Lowe, G.D.O., Lee, A.J., Rumley, A., Price, J.F., Fowkes, F.G.R., (1997). Blood viscosity and risk of cardiovascular events: the Edinburgh Artery Study. *British J. Haematol.* 96, 168-173.

[140] Rizza, S., Gigli, F., Galli, A., Micchelini, B., Lauro, D., Lauro, R., Federici, M., (2010). Adiponectin isoforms in elderly patients with or without coronary artery disease. *J. Am. Geriatr. Soc.* 58(4), 702–706.

[141] Bruckner, G., Fatty acids and cardiovascular disease. In: CK Chow, editor, Fatty acids in foods and their health implications. New York: Marcel Dekker, Inc; 2000; pp.843–863.

[142] Schaefer, E.J., (2002). Lipoproteins, nutrition, and heart disease. *Am. J. Clin. Nutr.* 75, 191–212.

[143] Siri-Tarino, P.W., Sun, Q., Hu, F.B., Krauss, R.M., (2010). Saturated fat, carbohydrate, and cardiovascular disease. *Am. J. Clin. Nutr.* 91, 502–509.

[144] Berglund, L., Lefevre, M., Ginsberg, H.N., Kris-Etherton, P.M., Elmer, P.J., Stewart, P.W., Ershow, A., Pearson, T.A., Dennis, B.H., Roheim, P.S., Ramakrishnan, R., Reed. R., Stewart, K., Phillips, K.M., (2007). Comparison of monounsaturated fat with carbohydrates as a replacement for saturated fat in subjects with a high metabolic risk profile: studies in the fasting and postprandial states. *Am. J. Clin. Nutr.* 86, 1611–1620.

[145] Pasini, E., Cargnoni, A., Condorelli, E., Marzo, A., Lisciani, R., Ferrari, R., (1992). Effect of prolonged treatment with propionyl-L-carnitine on erucic acid-induced myocardial dysfunction in rats. *Mol. Cell Biochem.* 112(2), 117-23.

[146] Simopoulos, A.P., (2002). The importance of the ratio of omega-6/omega-3 essential fatty acids. *Biomed. Pharmacother.* 56(8), 365-67.

[147] De Lorgeril, M., Salen, P., Paillard, F., Laporte, F., Boucher, F., de Leiris, J., (2002). Mediterranean diet and the French paradox: Two distinct biogeographic concepts for one consolidated scientific theory on the role of nutrition in coronary heart disease. *Cardiovasc. Res.* 54, 503–515.

[148] Sakata, Y., Shimokawa, H., (2013). Saturated fatty acid intake and cardiovascular risk. *Eur. Heart J.* 34(16), 1178-1180.

[149] ESFA., (2010). Scientific Opinion on Dietary Reference Values for fats, including saturated fatty acids, polyunsaturated fatty acids, monounsaturated fatty acids, trans fatty acids, and cholesterol. *EFSA J.* 8(3), 1461.

[150] Mali, P., Chou, B.K., Yen, J., Ye, Z., Zou, J., Dowey, S., Brodsky, R.A., Ohm, J.E., Yu, W., Baylin, S.B., Yusa, K., Bradley, A., Meyers, D.J., Mukherjee, C., Cole, P.A., Cheng, L., (2010). Butyrate Greatly Enhances Derivation of Human Induced Pluripotent Stem Cells by Promoting Epigenetic Remodeling and the Expression of Pluripotency-Associated Genes. *Stem Cells* 28(4), 713–720.

[151] Aggett, P.J., Iron. In: Erdman JW, Macdonald IA, Zeisel SH, eds. Present Knowledge in Nutrition. 10th ed. Washington, DC: Wiley-Blackwell; 2012; pp.506-20.

[152] Wessling-Resnick, M., Iron. In: Ross AC, Caballero B, Cousins RJ, Tucker KL, Ziegler RG, eds. Modern Nutrition in Health and Disease. 11th ed. Baltimore, MD: Lippincott Williams & Wilkins; 2014; pp.176-88.

[153] Hurrell, R., Egli, I., (2010). Iron bioavailability and dietary reference values. *Am. J. Clin. Nutr.* 91, 1461S-7S.

[154] USDA., (2014). Foods list, national nutrient database for standard reference Release 26. Available at: http://ndb.nal.usda.gov/ndb/foods/show/3834?fg=Beef+Products&man=&lfacet=&format=&count=&max=25&offset=&sort=&qlookup=spleen. Accessed 22 August 2014.

[155] PMFNB (Panel on Micronutrients, Food and Nutrition Board)., Dietary reference intakes for vitamin A, vitamin K, arsenic, boron, chromium, copper, iodine, iron, manganese, molybdenum, nickel, silicon, vanadium, and zinc. Washington, DC: National Academy Press; 2001; pp.9-1–78.

[156] Cheney, K., Gumbiner, C., Benson, B., Tenenbein, M., (1995). Survival after a severe iron poisoning treated with intermittent infusions of deferoxamine. *J. Toxicol. Clin. Toxicol.* 33(1), 61–6.

[157] Kremastinos, D.T., Farmakis, D., (2011). Iron overload cardiomyopathy in clinical practice. *Circulation* 124, 2253-63.

[158] Bacon, B.R., Adams, P.C., Kowdley, K.V., Powell, L.W., Tavill, A.S., (2011). Diagnosis and management of hemochromatosis: 2011 practice guideline by the American Association for the Study of Liver Diseases. *Hepatol.* 54, 328-43.

[159] Whitlock, E.P., Garlitz, B.A., Harris, E.L., Beil, T.L., Smith, P.R., (2006). Screening for hereditary hemochromatosis: a systematic review for the U.S. Preventive Services Task Force. *Ann. Intern. Med.* 145, 209-23.

[160] Murray-Kolbe, L.E., Beard, J., Iron. In: Coates PM, Betz JM, Blackman MR, et al., eds. Encyclopedia of Dietary Supplements. 2nd ed. London and New York: Informa Healthcare; 2010; pp.432-8.

[161] EFSA., (2004). Opinion of the scientific panel on dietetic products, nutrition and allergies on a request from the Commission related to the Tolerable upper intake level of iron (Request N EFSA-Q-2003-018; adopted on 19 October 2004). *EFSA J.* 125, 1-34.

[162] He, F.J., Li, J., MacGregor, G.A., (2013). Effect of longer-term modest salt reduction on blood pressure. *Cochrane Database Syst. Rev.* 4, CD004937. DOI: 10.1002/14651858. CD004937.pub2.

[163] Chobanian, A.V., Hill, M., (2000). National heart lung and blood institute workshop on sodium and blood pressure: A critical review of current scientific evidence. *Hypertens.* 35, 858–63.

[164] SACN (Scientific Advisory Committee on Nutrition)., Salt and health, SACN/SaltSub/03/02:1– 34. Norwich, UK: TSO (The Stationery Office); 2003.

[165] Schmieder, R.E., Messerli, F.H., (2000). Hypertension and the heart. *J. Hum. Hypertens.*14, 597–604.

[166] Safar, M.E., Thuilliez, C., Richard, V., Benetos, A., (2000). Pressure independent contribution of sodium to large artery structure and function in hypertension. *Cardiovasc. Res.* 46, 269–76.

[167] Simon, G., Illyes, G., (2000). High sodium diet induces structural vascular changes in rats without raising the blood pressure. *Am. J. Hypertens.* 13, 3001–10.

[168] Arcand, J., Ivanov, J., Sasson, A., Floras, V., Al-Hesayen, A., Azevedo, E.R., Mak, S., Allard, J.P., Newton, G.E., (2011). A high-sodium diet is associated with acute decompensated heart failure in ambulatory heart failure patients: a prospective follow-up study. Am. *J. Clin. Nutr.* 93, 332–37.

[169] Eap, C.B., Bochud, M., Elston, R.C., Bovet, P., Maillard, M.P., Nussberger, J., Schild, L., Shamlaye, C., Burnier, M., (2007). CYP3A5 and ABCB1 genes influence blood pressure and response to treatment, and their effect is modified by salt. *Hypertens.* 49, 1007–14.

[170] Kim, S.W., (2006). Hypernatemia: Successful treatment. *Electrol. Blood Press.* 4, 66-71.

[171] Ofran, Y., Lavi, D., Opher, D., Weiss, T.A., Elinav, E., (2004). Fatal voluntary salt intake resulting in the highest ever documented sodium plasma level in adults (255 mmol L^{-1}): a disorder linked to female gender and psychiatric disorders. *J. Intern. Med.* 256, 525–8.

[172] Institute of Medicine, Dietary reference intakes for water, potassium, sodium, chloride, and sulfate. Washington, D.C.: The National Academies Press; 2005.

[173] Mensah, G.A., Brown, D.W., (2007). An overview of cardiovascular disease burden in the United States. *Health Aff.* 26(1), 38-48.

[174] USDA and USDHHS (U.S. Department of Agriculture and U.S. Department of Health and Human Services), Dietary guidelines for Americans, 2010. 7th Edition. Washington, D.C., U.S.: Government Printing Office; 2010.

[175] De Wardener, H.E., He, F.J., Macgregor, G.A., (2004). Plasma sodium and hypertension. *Kidney Int.* 66, 2454–66.

[176] Weinberger, M.H., Fineberg, N.S., Fineberg, S.E., Weinberger, M., (2001). Salt sensitivity, pulse pressure, and death in normal and hypertensive humans. *Hypertens.* 37, 429–432.

[177] Stolarz-Skrzypek, K., Kuznetsova, T., Thijs, L., Tikhonoff, V., Seidlerová, J., Richart, T., Jin, Y., Olszanecka, A., Malyutina, S., Casiglia, E., Filipovský, J., Kawecka-Jaszcz, K., Nikitin, Y., Staessen, J.A., (2011). Fatal and nonfatal outcomes, incidence of hypertension, and blood pressure changes in relation to urinary sodium excretion. *J. Am. Med. Assoc.* 305(17), 1777-85.

[178] The Lancet, (2011). Salt and cardiovascular disease mortality. *Lancet.* 377(9778), 1626.

[179] Paterna, S., Gaspare, P., Fasullo, S., Sarullo, F.M., Di Pasquale, P., (2008). Normal-sodium diet compared with low-sodium diet in compensated congestive heart failure: Is sodium an old enemy or a new friend? *Clin. Sci. (Lond)* 114, 221–230.

[180] Thomas, M.C., Moran, J., Forsblom, C., Harjutsalo, V., Thorn, L., Ahola, A., Wadén, J., Tolonen, N., Saraheimo, M., Gordin, D., Groop, P.H., (2011). The association between dietary sodium intake, ESRD, and all-cause mortality in patients with type 1 diabetes. *Diab. Care* 34, 861–66.

[181] Mason, C.M., Doneen, A.L., (2012). Niacin: A Critical Component to the Management of Atherosclerosis Contemporary Management of Dyslipidemia to Prevent, Reduce, or Reverse Atherosclerotic Cardiovascular Disease. *J. Cardiovasc. Nursing* 27(Issue 4), 303–316.

[182] Brody, T., Nutritional Biochemistry, 2nd ed. San Diego: Academic Press; 1999.

[183] FNBIM (Food and Nutrition Board, Institute of Medicine), Dietary reference intakes: Thiamin, riboflavin, niacin, vitamin B_6, vitamin B_{12}, pantothenic acid, biotin, and choline. Washington, D.C.: National Academy Press; 1998; Pp.123-149.

[184] The AIM-HIGH Investigators., (2011). Niacin in Patients with Low HDL Cholesterol Levels Receiving Intensive Statin Therapy. *N. Engl. J. Med.* 365, 2255-67.

[185] Taylor, A.J., Lee, H.J., Sullenberger, L.E., (2006). The effect of 24 months of combination statin and extended-release niacin on carotid intima-media thickness: ARBITER 3. *Curr. Med. Res. Opin.* 22(11), 2243-50.

[186] Lavigne, P.M., Karas, R.H., (2013). The current state of niacin in cardiovascular disease prevention: a systematic review and meta-regression. *J. Am. Coll. Cardiol.* 61(4), 440-6.

[187] Goodman, L.S., Gilman, A., Brunton, L.L., Lazo, J.S., Parker, K.L., Goodman and Gilman's: the pharmacology basis of therapeutics. New York: McGrow-Hill; 2006.

[188] Mittal, M.K., Florin, T., Perrone, J., Delgado, J.H., Osterhoudt, K.C., (2007). Toxicity from the use of niacin to beat urine drug screening. *Ann. Emerg. Med.* 50, 587-590.

[189] Garg, R., Malinow, M., Pettinger, M., Upson, B., Hunninghake, D., (1999). Niacin treatment increases plasma homocyst(e)ine levels. *Am. Heart J.* 138, 1082-7.

[190] Garg, A., Grundy, S.M., (1990). Nicotinic acid as therapy for dyslipidemia in non-insulin-dependent diabetes mellitus. *J. Am. Med. Assoc.* 264(6), 723-6.

[191] Kamal-Bahl, S.J., Burke, T.A., Watson, D.J., Wentworth, C.E., (2008). Dosage, titration, and gaps in treatment with extended release niacin in clinical practice. *Curr. Med. Res. Opin.* 24(6), 1817-21.

[192] World Health Organization, Global status report on alcohol 2004. Geneva: WHO Library Cataloguing-in-Publication Data; 2004.

[193] Department of Mental Health and Substance Dependence, Non-communicable Diseases and Mental Health Cluster. International guide for monitoring alcohol consumption and related harm. Geneva (Switzerland): The World Health Organization; 2000; pp. 54. Available: http://whqlibdoc.who.int/hq /2000 /who _msd_msb _00.4.pdf (accessed 2012 Sept. 23)

[194] Liang, Y., Mente, A., Yusuf, S., Gao, P., Sleight, P., Zhu, J., Fagard, R., Lonn, E., Teo, K.K., (2012). Alcohol consumption and the risk of incident atrial fibrillation among people with cardiovascular disease. *CMAJ.* 184(16), E857-66.

[195] Adinoff, B., Bone, G.H., Linnoila, M., (1988). Acute ethanol poisoning and the ethanol withdrawal syndrome. *Med. Toxicol. Adverse Drug Exper.* 3(3), 172-96.

[196] Marmot, M.G., (2001). Alcohol and coronary heart disease. *Int. J. Epidemiol.* 30, 724-9.

[197] Thomson, A.D., Majumdar, S.K., The hazard to health from moderate drinking. In: MR Turner, editor, Nutrition and health: A perspective. Lancaster: MTP; 1982; pp.87-107.

[198] Kupari, M., Koskinen, P., Suokas, A., (1991). Left ventricular size, mass and function in relation to the duration and quantity of heavy drinking in alcoholics. *Am. J. Cardiol.* 67, 274-9.

[199] Kupari, M., Koskinen, P., Suokas, A., Ventil, M., (1990). Left ventricular filling impairment in asymptomatic chronic alcoholics. *Am. J. Cardiol.* 66, 1473-7.

[200] Fauchier, L., Babuty, D., Poret, P., Casset-Senon, D., Autret, M.L., Cosnay, P., Fauchier, J.P., (2000). Comparison of long-term outcome of alcoholic and idiopathic dilated cardiomyopathy. *Eur. Heart J.* 21, 306-14.

[201] Lazarevic, A.M., Nakatani, S., Neskovic, A.N., Marinkovic, J., Yasumura, Y., Stojicic, D., Miyatake, K., Bojic, M., Popovic, A.D., (2000). Early changes in left ventricular function in chronic asymptomatic alcoholics: Relation to the duration of heavy drinking. *J. Am. Coll. Cardiol.* 35, 1599-1606.

[202] Corrao, G., Rubbiati, L., Bagnardi, V., Zambon, A., Poikolainen, K., (2000). Alcohol and coronary heart disease: A meta-analysis. *Addiction* 95, 1505-23.

[203] Rossinen, J., Viitasalo, M., Partanen, J., Koskinen, P., Kupari, M., Nieminen, M.S., (1997). Effects of acute alcohol ingestion on heart rate variability in patients with documented coronary artery disease and stable angina pectoris. *Am. J. Cardiol.* 79, 487-91.

[204] Urbano-Márquez, A., Estruch, R., Fernández-Solá, J., Nicolás, J.M., Paré, J.C., Rubin, E., (1995). The greater risk of alcoholic cardiomyopathy and myopathy in women compared with men. *J. Am. Med. Assoc.* 274(2), 149-154.

[205] George, A., Figueredo, V.M., (2011). Alcoholic cardiomyopathy: A review. *J. Card. Fail.* 17(Iss.10), 844-849.

[206] Bing, R.J., (1978). Cardiac metabolsim: its contributions to alcoholic heart disease and myocardial failure. *Circulation* 58, 965-970.

[207] Trowell, H., (1972). Ischemic heart disease and dietary fiber. *Am. J. Clin. Nutr.* 25, 926-32.

[208] Truswell, AS., (2002). Cereal grains and coronary heart disease. *Eur. J. Clin. Nutr.* 56, 1-14.

[209] Van Horn, L., McCoin, M., Kris-Etherton, P.M., Burke, F., Carson, J.A., Champagne, C.M., Karmally, W., Sikand, G., (2008). The evidence for dietary prevention and treatment of cardiovascular disease. *J. Am. Diet. Assoc.* 108, 287-331.

[210] James, S.L., Muir, J.G., Curtis, S.L., Gibson, P.R., (2003). Dietary fibre: a roughage guide. *Intern. Med. J.* 33, 291-6.

[211] Lunn, J., Buttriss, J.L., (2007). Carbohydrates and dietary fibre. *Nutr. Bull.* 32, 21-64.

[212] Slavin, J.L., Martini, M.C., Jacobs, D.R., Marquart, L., (1999). Plausible mechanisms for the protectiveness of whole grains. *Am. J. Clin. Nutr.* 70(3 suppl), 459-63S.

[213] Jenkins, D.J., Wolever, T.M., Taylor, R.H., Barker, H., Fielden, H., Baldwin, J.M., Bowling, A.C., Newman, H.C., Jenkins, A.L., Goff, D.V., (1981). Glycemic index of foods: A physiologic basis for carbohydrate exchange. *Am. J. Clin. Nutr.* 34(3), 362-366.

[214] Brand-Miller, J., Foster-Powell, K., Colagiuri, S., The new glucose revolution. New York: Marlowe and Company; 2003.

[215] Foster-Powell, K., Holt, S.H.A., Brand-Miller, J.C., (2002) International table of glycaemic index and glycaemic load values: 2002. *Am. J. Clin. Nutr.* 76, 5-56.

[216] Jakobsen, M.U., Dethlefsen, C., Joensen, A.M., Stegger, J., Tjønneland, A., Schmidt, E.B., Overvad, K., (2010). Intake of carbohydrates compared with intake of saturated fatty acids and risk of myocardial infarction: importance of the glycemic index. *Am. J. Clin. Nutr.* 91, 1764–1768.

[217] Siri, P.W., Krauss, R.M., (2005). Influence of dietary carbohydrate and fat on LDL and HDL particle distributions. *Curr. Atherosc. Rep.* 7, 455–9.

[218] Parks, E.J., Hellerstein, M.K., (2000). Carbohydrate-induced hypertriacylglycerolemia: historical perspective and review of biological mechanisms. *Am. J. Clin. Nutr.* 71, 412–33.

[219] Carlson, L.A., Bottiger, L.E., (1972). Ischemic heart disease in relation to fasting values of plasma triglycerides and cholesterol. *Lancet.* 1, 865–8.

[220] Pereira, M.A., Liu, S., (2003). Types of carbohydrates and risk of cardiovascular disease. *J. Womens Health (Larchmt)* 12(2), 115-122.

[221] Sacks, F.M., Bray, G.A., Carey, V.J., Smith, S.R., Ryan, D.H., Anton, S.D., McManus, K., Champagne, C.M., Bishop, L.M., Laranjo, N., Leboff, M.S., Rood, J.C., de Jonge, L., Greenway, F.L., Loria, C.M., Obarzanek, E., Williamson, D.A., (2009). Comparison of weight-loss diets with different compositions of fat, protein, and carbohydrates. *N. Engl. J. Med.* 360(9), 859-73.

[222] Noakes, M., Keogh, J.B., Foster, P.R., Clifton, P.M., (2005). Effect of an energy-restricted, high-protein, low-fat diet relative to a conventional high-carbohydrate, low-fat diet on weight loss, body composition, nutritional status, and markers of cardiovascular health in obese women. *Am. J. Clin. Nutr.* 81(6), 1298-1306.

[223] Bantle, J.P., (2009). Dietary fructose and metabolic syndrome and diabetes. *J. Nutr.* 139, 1263S–1268S.

[224] Sharma, N., Okere, I.C., Barrows, B.R., Lei, B., Duda, M.K., Yuan, C.L., Previs, S.F., Sharov, V.G., Azimzadeh, A.M., Ernsberger, P., Hoit, B.D., Sabbah, H., Stanley, W.C., (2008). High-sugar diets increase cardiac dysfunction and mortality in hypertension compared to low-carbohydrate or high-starch diets. *J. Hypertens.* 26(7), 1402-10.

[225] Stirpe, F., Della Corte, E., Bonetti, E., Abbondanza, A., Abbati, A., De Stefano, F., (1970). Fructose-induced hyperuricaemia. *Lancet.* 2, 1310 –1.

[226] Stavric, B., Johnson, W.J., Clayman, S., Gadd, R.E., Chartrand, A., (1976). Effect of fructose administration on serum urate levels in the uricase inhibited rat. *Experientia* 32, 373– 4.

[227] WHO, Diet, nutrition and the prevention of chronic diseases: Report of a Joint WHO/FAO Expert Consultation. Geneva, Switzerland: World Health Organization; 2003.

[228] UNICEF/The Micronutrient Initiative, Vitamin and mineral deficiency: A global progress report. New York: UNICEF House; 2004.

[229] Moat, S.J., Lang, D., McDowell, I.F., Clarke, Z.L., Madhavan, A.K., Lewis, M.J., Goodfellow, J., (2004). Folate, homocysteine, endothelial function and cardiovascular disease. *J. Nutr. Biochem.* 15(2), 64-79.

[230] Qin, X., Li, J., Cui, Y., Liu, Z., Zhao, Z., Ge, J., Guan, D., Hu, J., Wang, Y., Zhang, F., Xu, X., Wang, X., Xu, X., Huo, Y., (2012). MTHFR C677T and MTR A2756G polymorphisms and the homocysteine lowering efficacy of different doses of folic acid in hypertensive Chinese adults. *Nutr. J.* 11, 2-8.

[231] de Bree, A., van Dusseldorp, M., Brouwer, I.A., van het Hof, K.H., Steegers-Theunissen, R.P., (1997). Folate intake in Europe: recommended, actual and desired intake. *Eur. J. Clin. Nutr.* 51(10), 643–60.

[232] Wald, D.S., Bishop, L., Wald, N.J., Law, M., Hennessy, E., Weir, D., McPartlin, J., Scott, J., (2001). Randomized trial of folic acid supplementation and serum homocysteine levels. *Arch. Intern. Med.* 161, 695–700.

[233] Lotto, V., Choi, S.W., Friso, S., (2011). Vitamin B_6: a challenging link between nutrition and inflammation in CVD. *Brit. J. Nutr.* 106, 183–195.

[234] Leklem, J.E., (1990). Vitamin B_6: a status report. *J. Nutr.* 120(Suppl.11), 1503–7.

[235] Selhub, J., Jacques, P.F., Dallal, G., Choumenkovitch, S., Rogers, G., (2008). The use of blood concentrations of vitamins and their respective functional indicators to define folate and vitamin B12 status. *Food Nutr. Bull.* 29(Suppl.2), S67-73.

[236] Selhub, J., Jacques, P.F., Wilson, P.W., Rush, D., Rosenberg, I.H., (1993). Vitamin status and intake as primary determinants of homocysteinemia in an elderly population. *J. Am. Med. Assoc.* 270, 2693-8.

[237] van Oijen, M.G.H., Laheij, R.J.F., Jansen, J.B.M.J., Verheugt, F.W.A., (2007). The predictive value of vitamin B_{12} concentrations and hyperhomocysteinaemia for cardiovascular disease. *Neth. Heart J.* 15, 291-4.

[238] Debreceni, B., Debreceni, L., (2014). The role of homocysteine-lowering B-vitamins in the primary prevention of cardiovascular disease. *Cardiovasc. Ther.* 32(3), 130-8.

[239] Bønaa, K.H., Njølstad, I., Ueland, P.M., Schirmer, H., Tverdal, A., Steigen, T., Wang, H., Nordrehaug, J.E., Arnesen, E., Rasmussen, K., (2006). Homocysteine lowering and cardiovascular events after acute myocardial infarction. *N. Eng. J. Med.* 354, 1578-88.

[240] Coultate, T.D., FOOD: The Chemistry of Its Components, 2nd edition. Royal Society of Chemistry, Cambridge; 1989; pp. 287-288.

[241] DeLuca, H., (2004). Overview of General physiological tenures and function of vitamin D. *Am. J. Clin. Nutr.* 80, 16895–16965.

[242] Gruber, M., Hu, C.J., Johnson, R.S., Brown, E.J., Keith, B., Simon, M.C., (2007). Acute postnatal ablation of Hif-2alpha results in anemia. *Proc. Natl. Acad. Sci. USA* 104, 2301-2306.

[243] Institute of Medicine, Dietary reference intakes for calcium and vitamin D. Washington, D.C: National Academies Press; 2011.

[244] Dietary Reference Intakes for Calcium and Vitamin D. Report of the Institute of Medicine of the National Academies; November 30, 2010.

[245] Brøndum-Jacobsen, P., Benn, M., Jensen, G.B., Nordestgaard, B.G., (2012). 25-Hydroxyvitamin D levels and risk of ischemic heart disease, myocardial infarction, and early death: population-based study and meta-analyses of 18 and 17 studies. *Arterioscler. Thromb. Vasc. Biol.* 32, 2794-2802.

[246] Holick, M.F., (2007). Vitamin D deficiency. *N. Engl. J. Med.* 357, 266–281.

[247] Hyppönen, E., Läärä, E., Reunanen, A., Järvelin, M.R., Virtanen, S.M., (2001). Intake of vitamin D and risk of type 1 diabetes: a birth-cohort study. *Lancet.* 358, 1500–3.

[248] von Hurst, P.R., Stonehouse, W., Coad, J., (2010). Vitamin D supplementation reduces insulin resistance in South Asian women living in New Zealand who are insulin resistant and vitamin D deficient: a random-ized, placebo-controlled trial. *Br. J. Nutr.* 103, 549–55.

[249] Artaza, J.N., Mehrotra, R., Norris, K.C., (2009). Vitamin D and the cardiovascular system. *Clin. J. Am. Soc. Nephrol.* 4, 1515–22.

[250] Lavie, C.J., Lee, J.H., Milani, R.V., (2011). Vitamin D and cardiovascular disease: Will it live up to its hype? *J. Am. Coll. Cardiol.* 58, 1547–56.

[251] Wong, M.S.K., Leisegang, M.S., Kruse, C., Vogel, J., Schürmann, C., Dehne, N., Weigert, A., Herrmann, E., Brüne, B., Shah, A.M., Steinhilber, D., Offermanns, S., Carmeliet, G., Badenhoop, K., Schröder, K., Brandes, R.P., (2014). Vitamin D promotes vascular regeneration. *Circulation* 130, 976-986.

[252] Elin, R.J., (1988). Magnesium metabolism in health and disease. *Dis. Mon.* 34, 161–218.

[253] Swaminathan, R., (2003). Magnesium metabolism and its disorders. *Clin. Biochem. Rev.* 24, 47–66.
[254] Saris, N.E., Mervaala, E., Karppanen, H., Khawaja, J.A., Lewenstam, A., (2000). Magnesium. An update on phys-iological, clinical and analytical aspects. *Clin. Chim. Acta* 294, 1–26.255.
[255] Aikawa, J.K., Magnesium: Its Biological Significance. Boca Ra-ton, FL: CRC Press; 1981.
[256] Elin, R.J., (1988). Magnesium metabolism in health and disease. *Dis. Mon.* 34, 161–218.
[257] Wacker, W., Magnesium and Man. Cambridge, MA: Havard University Press; 1980; pp.1–184.
[258] Shechter, M., Merz, C.N., Paul-Labrador, M., Meisel, S.R., Rude, R.K., Molloy, M.D., Dwyer, J.H., Shah, P.K., Kaul, S., (1999). Oral magnesium supplementation inhibits platelet-dependent thrombosis in patients with coronary artery disease. *Am. J. Cardiol.* 84, 152–156.
[259] Altura, B.M., Altura, B.T., (1985). New perspectives on the role of mag-nesium in the pathophysiology of the cardiovascular system. I. Clinical aspects. *Magnesium* 4, 226–244.
[260] Faboya, O.O., (1985). Chlorophyll changes in some green leafy vegetables during cooking. *J. Sci. Food Agr.* 36(8), 740–744.
[261] Graham, L., Caesar, J., Burgen, A., (1960). Gastrointestinal absorption and excretion of Mg^{28} in man. *Metab.* 9, 646-659.
[262] Champagne, C.M., (2008). Magnesium in hypertension, cardiovascular disease, metabolic syndrome, and other conditions: A review. *Nutr. Clin. Pract.* 23(2), 142-51.
[263] Wong, E.T., Rude, R.K., Singer, F.R., Shaw, S.T., (1983). A high prevalence of hypomagnesemia and hypermagnesemia in hospitalized patients. *J. Clin. Pathol.* 79, 348–352.
[264] Hashizume, N., Mori, M., (1990). An analysis of hypermagnesemia and hypomagnesemia. *Jap. J. Med.* 29, 368–372.
[265] Guerrero-Romero, F., Tamez-Perez, H.E., González-González, G., Salinas-Martínez, A.M., Montes-Villarreal, J., Treviño-Ortiz, J.H., Rodríguez-Morán, M., (2004). Oral magnesium supplementation improves insulin sensitivity in non-diabetic subjects with insulin resistance. A double-blind placebo-controlled randomized trial. *Diab. Metab.* 30, 253–8.
[266] Chernow, B., Bamberger, S., Stoiko, M., Vadnais, M., Mills, S., Hoellerich, V., Warshaw, A.L., (1989). Hypomagnesemia in patients in postoperative intensive care. *Chest.* 95, 391–7.
[267] Whang, R., Ryder, K.W., (1990). Frequency of hypomagnesemia and hypermagnesemia. Requested vs routine. *J. Am. Med. Assoc.* 263, 3063–4.
[268] Jahnen-Dechent, W., Ketteler, M., (2012). Magnesium basics. *Clin. Kidney J.* 5(Suppl.1), i3–i14.
[269] Golzarian, J., Scott, H.W., Richards, W.O., (1994). Hypermagnesemia-induced paralytic ileus. *Dig. Dis. Sci.* 39, 1138-42.
[270] Berns, A.S., Kollmeyer, K.R., (1976). Magnesium-induced bradycardia. *Ann. Intern. Med.* 85, 760-1.

Chapter 4

Consumption of Trans-Fatty Acids

According to the bonds existing in the carbon chain (or backbone), fatty acids are usually classified as two groups: saturated and unsaturated fatty acids. There are only single bonds in the carbon chain of saturated fatty acids. The single bond can rotate freely and therefore no structural isomer exists. In contrast, there is at least one double bond in the carbon chain of unsaturated fatty acids. If the two hydrogen atoms take up positions on, or the carbon chain extends from the opposite sides of the double bond in the carbon chain of an unsaturated fatty acid, it is a trans fatty acid (TFA) (Figure 9). If the two hydrogen atoms take up positions on, or the carbon chain extends from the same sides of the double bond in the carbon chain of an unsaturated fatty acid, it is a cis fatty acid. A TFA has a bent carbon chain whereas a cis fatty acid has a straighter carbon chain. A fat contains fatty acids with trans configurations would have a physical properties (i.e. semi-solid at room temperature) similar to that of a saturated fat. One or more trans double bonds may be found in a trans lipid (fat) molecule. Such a subtle difference of the structure results in the very different healthy effect of TFAs from other unsaturated fatty acids.

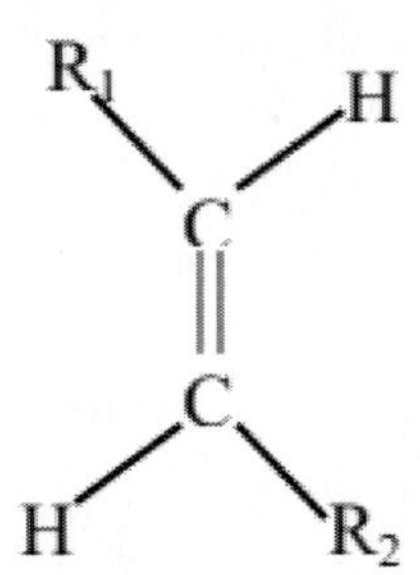

Figure 9. Structure diagram of trans fatty acids.

Dietary Sources of Trans Fatty Acids

Naturally occurring *trans* fats are mainly found in meats and dairy products from cows, sheeps, and other ruminants, which result from bacteria actions in the ruminant stomach. Reports on the concentration of *trans* fats in these kinds of food resources by different authors seem to be inconsistent. It was reported that *trans* fats account for about 5% of ruminant fats

[1] while it was also reported that 2–5% and as high as 8% *trans* fats in the total fats in most ruminant-based foods for example beef and dairy products, and in lamb meats, respectively [2]. Trans-fat content in the oils of milk is generally less than 2.5%. The naturally occurring *trans* fats found in the rumen of ruminants are identified to be vaccenic acid and conjugated linoleic acid. There are two double bonds in the carbon chain of conjugated linoleic acid. One double bond is in the *trans* configuration and another is in *cis*. It should be noted that human milk may contain *trans* fats with varying amounts that rely on the maternal intake of *trans* fats. The content (% of total fats) of *trans* fats in human milk was reported to be 7% in the United States and Canada, 4% in Germany, 2% in France, and 1% in Spain [3].

Their content in margarine (or butter) and other partially hydrogenated oils (or fats) could be as high as 20-60% (w/w) [4] whereas no *trans* fats would form when the double bonds are fully hydrogenated. Scientists studied on the development of techniques for the hydrogenation avoiding the side effect of forming *trans* fats. It was found that the content of *trans* fats was greatly affected by the pressure during hydrogenation. The hydrogenation of soy oils at 200 psi (1400 kPa) and 140°C - 170°C heating condition resulted in ca. 17% TFAs by weight, comparing with ca. 40% produced by employing the standard 20 psi (140 kPa) hydrogenating process at the same temperature range. When the hydrogenated fats produced at the high pressure are mixed with liquid soybean oils unhydrogenated, the content of *trans* fats in the margarine obtained is 5- 6%. This level was allowed to claim as the margarine free of *trans* fat according the labeling requirements [5] still effective in 2005 in USA [6] whereas it has now been recommended that the consumption of *trans* fat should be as low as possible [7]. The regulation of the hydrogenating time or the hydrogenating temperature could also change the concentration of formed *trans* fats in a product. It is also possible to form *trans* fats when refining vegetable oils or deep-frying by using the vegetable oils over long periods at high temperatures though the amounts formed may be very small (0.2-1% total fats) [2].

Naturally occurring *trans* fats are reported to contribute to about 0.5% of total energy intakes [8]. The percentage of *trans* fats from processed foods contributing total energy intakes varies with the variation of amount of hydrogenated fats added and their *trans* fat content.

Many processed foods such as deep-fried fast foods, bakery products, packaged snack foods, margarines, and crackers may contain significant amounts of *trans* fats if partially hydrogenated fats are added to these foods. Furthermore, some restaurants may produce fast foods with abundant amounts of *trans* fats [9]. People who frequently eat this kind of fast foods or who are not used to consume foods with the presence of fewer hydrogenated fats should ingest larger quantities of *trans* fats.

Trans Fatty Acids and CVDs

The research on the adverse effect of *trans* fats on human health is attracting more and more attentions, which is continuing nowadays. Scientific evidences consistently indicate that the ingestion of TFAs increases the risk of CVDs. It was reported that the ingestion of certain amount of TFAs has the potential of resulting in many health problems throughout the entire lifetime [10]. Furthermore, long term prospective cohort studies showed that a TFA intake, irrespective of source, was positively associated with CVDs [11].

Initially, one theory reported in the literature believed that the enzyme, lipase in the human body, acts only on fats with the *cis* configuration and the metabolism of those with the *trans* configuration cannot take place. However, this theory has been proved to be not correct by the understanding of the fact that the metabolism of *trans* fats actually takes place in the human body and competitively restrains the metabolism of other fatty acids [12]. For example, it was found that the metabolism of long-chain polyunsaturated fatty acids was abnormal possibly due to the adverse effect of TFAs [13]. The body's capacity of metabolizing essential fatty acids (ω-6, ω-3) can be interfered by the presence of *trans* fats, which would result in the variations of composition of fatty acids that comprise phospholipids in the main artery of the heart (the aorta), and therefore lift the possibility of developing coronary heart diseases [14].

The occurrence of Type 2 Diabetes was found to be at least partially associated with the ingestion of *trans* fats [15] though more investigations are needed to illustrate the exact mechanism for the promotion of diabetes by *trans* fats. More and more people are increasingly concerned about increases in the risk of Type 2 Diabetes caused by increases in the ingestion of *trans* fats [2]. However, greater efforts are necessary for reaching consensus [8]. For example, one report stated that people who had the higher ingestion of *trans* fats were found to have the higher risk of developing diabetes [16]. Furthermore, *trans* fats was reported to be involved in the development of insulin resistance since the impairment of post-insulin receptor binding signal transduction was observed [17]. On the other hand, another report described that the risk of diabetes was found to be not associated with the ingestion of *trans* fats when such other factors as body weight index and total fats ingested were taken into consideration [18]. The ingestion of *trans* fats may be associated with obesity. Some scientific studies showed that the ingestion of *trans* fats with a similar caloric intake to other fats had the potential of increasing abdominal fats and weight gains [17]. The authors found that the diet containing *trans* fats resulted in 7.2 % increases in body weight whereas that containing mono-unsaturated fats only caused 1.8% increases in body weight by carrying out a 6-year experiment on monkeys. The same authors also concluded that TFAs promoted the intra-abdominal deposition of fats, even without the presence of excessive calories. It seems that it is quite difficult to find more studying results of supporting the conclusion about the association of *trans* fats with obesity in the literature. More studies would be necessary for achieving a strong scientific consensus relating to the association of obesity with *trans* fats (as an independent factor of causing weight gains). In addition to the scientific evidences connecting *trans* fats and diabetes or obesity that are risk factors of CVDs mentioned above, there are also experimental results that illustrate the direct association of *trans* fats with coronary heart diseases or other risk factors for CVDs. For example, the involvement of high ingestion of *trans* fats in high blood pressure (a great risk for CVDs) and other biomarkers of developing CVDs should not be ignored also. Short term controlled trials found that a TFA intake was associated with CHDs, adverse lipid metabolism, systemic inflammation, and endothelial dysfunction that are positively associated with CVDs [8].

Trans Fats and Coronary Heart Disease

The increased ingestion of *trans* fats was found to primarily result in an increased risk of a coronary heart disease (CHD) [2]. The ingestion of *trans* fats was reported to be associated with more than 30,000 cardiac deaths in the United States, which was estimated in 1994 [19]. It was estimated that deaths due to cardiac diseases associated with the ingestion of *trans* fats increased to 100,000 by 2006 [20]. A strong and reliable association of *trans* fat ingestion with the morbidity of CHD was stated by authors who published a comprehensive review paper including substantial amounts of experimental results in 2006 in the New England Journal of Medicine. The authors concluded in their paper that "On a per-calorie basis, *trans* fats appear to increase the risk of CHD more than any other macronutrient, conferring a substantially increased risks at low levels of consumption (1 to 3% of total energy intake)" [8]. The report published by Hu and others indicated the major evidence of the reliable association of *trans* fats with CHDs. A cohort study was described in the report, which started up in 1976 and involved 120,000 female subjects. In this Nurses' Health Study, the authors found 900 individuals with coronary problems during 14 years of follow-up. They concluded that every 2% elevation of *trans* fat calories ingested (replacing saccharide calories) resulted in approximately 2 times increases in the risk of CHD whereas every 5% elevation of saturated fat calories (replacing saccharide calories) only caused a 17% elevation of the risk of CHD. They also found that substituting *trans* unsaturated fats or saturated fats by *cis* (unhydrogenated) unsaturated fats resulted in greater decreases in the risk of CHD, compared to replacing them isocalorically with saccharides [21]. In addition, they reported the beneficial effects of decreasing the ingestion of *trans* fats. They stated that 2% of dietary energy from non-*trans* unsaturated fats instead of *trans* fats resulted in 53% decreases in the risk of CHD whereas 5% of dietary energy from non-trans unsaturated fats instead of saturated fats just achieved about 43% decreases in the risk of CHD. It was also reported that the ingestion of *trans* fats was associated with the mortality of CHD since the ingestion of polyunsaturated fats instead of *trans* fats greatly reduced the mortality of CHD [2,22].

Effect on Blood Lipid Profile

Blood tests are usually accepted for estimating the risk of CVDs in individuals. One report published in 2003 compared the influence of having meals containing abundant amounts of *trans* and *cis* fats on the lipid profile in the blood by carrying out a randomized crossover study. The authors stated that the meal containing *trans* fats resulted in 28% increases in cholesteryl ester transfer and enriched lipoprotein levels in apolipoprotein(a) (the positive association of Lp(a) level with CVDs reported in the literature [23]), as compared to the meal containing *cis* fats [24]. It should be however noted that the determination of blood cholesterols, especially a HDLC/LDLC or TC ratio, is more widely accepted than other methods.

Some outcomes of the adverse lipid metabolism induced by a TFA intake include increases in the levels of apoprotein (Apo) B (the main protein for forming LDL) and cholesteryl ester transfer protein (the main enzyme for transferring cholesterol esters from HDL to LDL and VLDL), the cellular accumulation or the secretion of free cholesterols or cholesterol esters by hepatocytes, and the rate of ApoA-I (the main protein for forming HDL) catabolism, and decreases in ApoA-I levels and the rate of LDL ApoB-100 catabolism, compared with the intake of the same amount of calories from saturated or *cis*-unsaturated fats.

These outcomes cause increases in LDLCs, decreases in HDLCs [25], and subsequent decreases in the HDLC/LDLC or TC ratio (also see Chapter 2 Cholesterol mentioned above). The ingestion of *trans* fats elevates the concentration of LDLC levels in the blood like what saturated fats do, but significantly reduces the concentration of HDLC levels in the blood. It has almost been guaranteed that the net decrease in the HDLC/LDLC ratio caused by the ingestion of *trans* fats is about two times of those caused by saturated fats [25-27]. (Higher ratios are better for reducing the risk of CVDs.) For example, it was reported that the elevation of plasma LDLC or lipoprotein (a) concentrations and decreasee in HDLC levels caused by TFAs were indicated by several clinical investigations [28]. A 2008 Dutch meta-analysis published in 2010 stated that all *trans* fats, regardless of originating from artificial or natural food resources, equally increase LDLC levels and reduce HDLC concentrations in the blood [29].

There are also other outcomes of the adverse lipid metabolism, such as increases in the levels of Lp(a) lipoproteins and blood triglycerides, and decreases in the size of LDL particles. Furthermore, TFAs intake reduces triglyceride uptake and the esterification of newly synthesized cholesterols, and increases the production of free fatty acids in adipocytes.

Causing Inflammation

The biomarkers of inflammation include the increased levels of TNF-α, IL-6, CRP, TNF receptors, and monocyte chemoattractant protein 1 that play roles in developing CVDs. The increase in these biomarkers may be due to the modulation of monocyte and macrophage responses in humans by TFAs. The determination of the blood CRP (one of cytokine) may also be a good way to estimate the risk of CVDs in individuals. The CRP is a cell-signaling cytokine. The test of this cytokine might be more powerful than that of others, which is however still a hot topic of investigations [2]. It was reported in the literature that the highest quartile of ingestion of *trans* fats resulted in 73% increases in the blood CRP, as compared to the lowest quartile of ingestion of *trans* fats [30]. The ingestion of foods containing *trans* fats would increase their concentration in membranes in patients with established CVDs and the elevated level of membrane *trans* fats was found to be independently involved in activating systemic inflammatory responses (for example, the substantially elevated concentrations of monocyte chemoattractant protein 1, TNF receptors, TNF-α, and IL-6) [31]. An investigation into women overweighted again indicated that the increased ingestion of *trans* fats resulted in the elevated concentrations of CRP and IL-6, and the activities of the TNF system [30]. Another investigation into women also showed that the increased ingestion of TFAs was involved in the elevated activities of TNF-α system while the elevated concentrations of IL-6 and CRP were also observed in those with a higher body weight [32].

Randomized and controlled tests have also indicated the inflammation effects of *trans* fats. It was found that the diet containing soybean-margarine (6.7% of energy contributed by TFAs) increased the level of TNF-α and IL-6 in cultured mononuclear cells in subjects with hypercholesterolemia after one month trial, as compared to the diet containing soybean-oils (only 0.6% of energy contributed by TFAs) though the level of IL-1β was quite similar [33]. By comparing to oleic acid, another investigation showed that TFAs (contributing to 8% of energy in the diet) greatly elevated the concentrations of CRP and IL-6 in the blood after a trial for 5 weeks [34]. These investigations indicated that the inflammation impacts of TFAs were quite similar to those of saturated fats.

It has been stated that the inflammation without the presence of other risk factors independently increases the risk of heart failure, diabetes, sudden deaths from cardiac causes and atherosclerosis [35-38]. The inflammation may be just a part of the adverse impacts of TFAs on the health of the cardiovascular system. For instance, the increased level of CRP resulted from the ingestion of a diet containing *trans* fats (accounting for 2.1% of total energy ingestion) would be able to elevate CVD risks of about 30%, as compared to that containing *trans* fats accounting for 0.9% of total energy ingestion [30], basing on the positive relation of the risk of CVDs and CRP concentrations [8,39].

Causing Endothelial Dysfunction

The biomarkers of endothelial dysfunction include the increased levels of SICAM 1, SVCAM 1, and E-selectin. These markers of endothelial dysfunction are positively associated with TFA intakes. In other words, the ingestion of *trans* fats is likely to result in endothelial dysfunction. For example, it was reported that an increased ingestion of TFAs significantly elevated the concentration of such biomarkers as SICAM 1, SVCAM 1, and E-selectin after other risk factors were adjusted [30].

The result of the elevated concentrations of E-selectin mentioned above was analogous to that of a randomized test (i.e. isocalorically oleic acids or saccharides with *trans* fats) [34]. The development of arterial plaque involves the elevation of these soluble cell adhesion molecules on the vascular endothelium.

Another marker of endothelial dysfunction is a reduction in brachial artery flow-mediated vasodilatation. It was reported that the ingestion of certain amount of TFAs resulted in the impairment of endothelial function, i.e. brachial artery flow-mediated vasodilatation reduced by 29%, as compared to the consumption of saturated fats [40].

Nitric oxide (NO) generally acts as a vascular homeostatic agent and vasodilator. A decrease in the synthesis or function of NO is believed to be one of markers of endothelial dysfunction. A decline in the bioavailability or levels of NO significantly elevates the possibility of development of hypertension or atherosclerosis. The intake of TFAs greatly decreases the synthesis and bioavailability of NO in endothelial cells [41].

Promotion of Other Risk Factors for CVDs

TFA intakes may also promote other risk factors for CVDs, such as the reduced activity of serum paraoxonase (an enzyme that is closely associated with HDLC), the impaired postprandial activity of tissue plasminogen activator, and insulin resistance.

Furthermore, some case-control studies showed that TFA intakes increased TFA levels in adipose tissues and red blood cells. The increased TFA levels in adipose tissues may increase the incidence of deaths caused by CHDs [42]. Also, total TFA levels in red blood cells were found to increase the risk of cardiac arrest (sudden death) [43].

Dietary Guidelines and Regulations

According to the contexts that are described above in this chapter, it is therefore believed that the recommended intake of TFAs being kept less than 1% of the total energy intake should be important [44]. All guidelines should be based on the scientific consensus of believing the adverse impacts of TFAs on human health and the increasing wide use of vegetable oils that are partially hydrogenated (e.g. directly eaten with a daily diet or added to processed foods) since 100 years ago (particularly, the later half of the 20th century) [9].

Literature search indicates that there are various guidelines proposed in different countries or by different organizations. For example, manufacturers in Australia have actually produced margarine with the avoidance of *trans* fats since 1996 though no requirement for separately showing *trans* fats in addition to a total fat content is currently assigned by Australia's food labeling laws [45]. In Denmark, *trans* fats in dietary oils or fats are not allowed to be higher than 2% by regulations (or laws) and this regulatory practice leads to the possibility of "far lower" than 1 g daily consumption of *trans* fats that are industrially produced [46]. It is hypothetically estimated that a 50% reduction in the mortality of ischemic heart diseases is associated with the Danish government's efforts for more than 20 years to reduce the daily ingestion of *trans* fats from 6 g to 1 g [47]. In U.K., an editorial published in 2010 in British Medical Journal suggested the virtual removal of *trans* fats from foods [48]. In the same year, the British National Institute for Health and Clinical Excellence supported this editorial suggestion [49]. And also, *trans* fats were suggested to be listed in food labels as cholesterols and saturated fats [50]. In USA, the National Academy of Sciences (NAS) has stated that the safe intake level of and adequate data for recommending daily upper tolerable limit for *trans* fat intakes are not established. The reason for this may be that any incremental elevation of *trans* fat consumption results in the elevation of CHD risks [51]. Despite all that, the requirement of eliminating *trans* fats from daily foods or diets has not been included in the NAS dietary recommendations. This is based on the fact that many animal foods inevitably contain trace amounts of *trans* fats, and therefore the processes of eliminating it from ordinary foods might result in the contamination of undesirables and the destruction or imbalance of nutrients if no appropriate nutritional fortification is implemented. Therefore, it has been suggested by the NAS that the intake of TFAs be as low as possible with the consumption of a diet that is nutritionally adequate [51]. World Health Organization suggested that the consumption of *trans* fats be controlled to the level <1% of total energy ingestion with the purpose of balancing the goals of public health [2].

It should also be noted that the US National Dairy Council has argued that the *trans* fats originated from animal food resources are quite different from those produced by the partial hydrogenation of oils, and seem to have no similar adverse impacts on cardiovascular health [52]. Furthermore, other investigations appear to indicate a positive effect of *trans* fats (e.g. conjugated linoleic acid) originating from animal food resources on human health. It was reported that the *cis*-9, *trans*-11 form of conjugated linoleic acid was able to help against inflammation, decrease the risk of CVDs, and prevent cancer [53,54]. Controversially, the limitation of adverse effects of *trans* fats originating from ruminant products may result from the low intake, compared to artificial ones [8].

References

[1] Sun, Q., (2008). Trans Fat and Cardiovascular Disease. *N. Am. J. Med. Sci.* 1(1), 34-35.

[2] L'Abbé, M.R., Brown, S., Report of the Trans Fat Task Force Submitted to the Minister of Health. Published by authority of the Minister of Health, Canada; 2006. Available at: www.healthcanada.ca/transfat

[3] Innis, S.M., King, D.J., (1999). Trans fatty acids in human milk are inversely associated with concentrations of essential all cis n-6 and n-3 fatty acids and determine trans, but not n-6 and n-3, fatty acids in plasma lipids of breast-fed infants. *Am. J. Clin. Nutr.* 70(3), 383–390.

[4] Mozaffarian, D., Clarke, R., (2009). Quantitative effects on cardiovascular risk factors and coronary heart disease risk of replacing partially hydrogenated vegetable oils with other fats and oils. *Eur. J. Clin. Nutr.* 63, S22–S33.

[5] FDA., Regulation: 21 CFR 101.9 (c)(2)(ii). 21 CFR Part 101. Food labeling; trans fatty acids in nutrition labeling; consumer research to consider nutrient content and health claims and possible footnote or disclosure statements; final rule and proposed rule. National Archives and Records Administration; 2003. Available at: http://www.gpo.gov/fdsys/pkg/CFR-2010-title21-vol2/pdf/CFR-2010-title21-vol2-sec101-9.pdf

[6] Eller, F.J., List, G.R., Teel, J.A., Steidley, K.R., Adlof, R.O., (2005). Preparation of spread oils meeting U.S. Food and Drug Administration labeling requirements for trans fatty acids via pressure-controlled hydrogenation. *J. Agr. Food Chem.* 53(15), 5982–5984.

[7] USDA and USDHHS (U.S. Department of Agriculture and U.S. Department of Health and Human Services)., Dietary guidelines for Americans, 2010. 7th Edition. Washington, D.C., U.S.: Government Printing Office; 2010.

[8] Mozaffarian, D., Katan, M.B., Ascherio, A., Stampfer, M.J., Willett, W.C., (2006). Trans fatty acids and cardiovascular disease. *N. Engl. J. Med.* 354, 1601-13.

[9] Valenzuel, A., Morgado, N., (1999). Trans fatty acid isomers in human health and in the food industry. *Biol. Res.* 32(4), DOI: 10.4067/S0716-97601999000400007

[10] Menaa, F., Menaa, A., Menaa, B., Tréton, J., (2013). Trans-fatty acids, dangerous bonds for health? *Eur. J. Nutr.* 52(4), 1289–302.

[11] Laake, I., Pedersen, J.I., Selmer, R., Kirkhus, B., Lindman, A.S., Tverdal, A., Veierød, M.B., (2012). A prospective study of intake of trans-fatty acids from ruminant fat, partially hydrogenated vegetable oils, and marine oils and mortality from CVD. *Brit. J. Nutr.*108, 743–754.

[12] Booyens, J., Louwrens, C.C., Katzeff, I.E., (1988). The role of unnatural dietary trans and cis unsaturated fatty acids in the epidemiology of coronary artery disease. *Med. Hypotheses*. 25(3), 175–82.

[13] Mozaffarian, D., Katan, M.B., Ascherio, A., Stampfer, M.J., Willett, W.C., (2003). Influence of trans fatty acids on infant and fetus development. *Acta Microbiol. Polon.* 52, 67–74.

[14] Kummerow, F.A.1., Zhou, Q., Mahfouz, M.M., Smiricky, M.R., Grieshop, C.M., Schaeffer, D.J., (2004). Trans fatty acids in hydrogenated fat inhibited the synthesis of the polyunsaturated fatty acids in the phospholipid of arterial cells. *Life Sci.* 74(22), 2707–23.

[15] Riserus, U., (2006). Trans fatty acids, insulin sensitivity and type 2 diabetes. *Scand. J. Food Nutr.* 50(4), 161–165.

[16] Hu, F.B., van Dam, R.M., Liu, S., (2001). Diet and risk of Type II diabetes: the role of types of fat and carbohydrate. *Diabetologia* 44(7), 805–817.

[17] Kavanagh, K., Jones, K.L., Sawyer, J., Kelley, K., Carr, J.J., Wagner, J.D., Rudel, L.L., (2007). Trans Fat Diet Induces Abdominal Obesity and Changes in Insulin Sensitivity in Monkeys. *Obesity (Silver Spring)* 15(7), 1675-1684.

[18] van Dam, R.M., Stampfer, M., Willett, W.C., Hu, F.B., Rimm, E.B., (2002). Dietary fat and meat intake in relation to risk of type 2 diabetes in men. *Diabetes Care* 25(3), 417–424.

[19] Willett, W., Ascherio, A., (1994). Trans Fatty Acids: Are the Effects Only Marginal? *Circulation* 84(5), 722–724.

[20] Zaloga, G.P., Harvey, K.A., Stillwell, W., Siddiqui, R., (2006). Trans Fatty Acids and Coronary Heart Disease. *Nutr. Clin. Pract.* 21(5), 505–512.

[21] Hu, F.B., Stampfer, M.J., Manson, J.E., Rimm, E., Colditz, G.A., Rosner, B.A., Hennekens, C.H., Willett, W.C., (1997). Dietary fat intake and the risk of coronary heart disease in women. *N. Engl. J. Med.* 337(21), 1491–1499.

[22] Oh, K., Hu, F.B., Manson, J.E., Stampfer, M.J., Willett, W.C., (2005). Dietary fat intake and risk of coronary heart disease in women: 20 years of follow-up of the nurses' health study. *Am. J. Epidemiol.* 161(7), 672–679.

[23] Brown, S.A., Morrisett, J.D., Boerwinkle, E., Hutchinson, R., Patsch, W., (1993). The relation of lipoprotein[a] concentrations and apolipoprotein[a] phenotypes with asymptomatic atherosclerosis in subjects of the Atherosclerosis Risk in Communities (ARIC) Study. *Arterioscler. Thromb.* 13, 1558-1566.

[24] Gatto, L.M., Sullivan,D.R., Samman, S., (2003). Postprandial effects of dietary trans fatty acids on apolipoprotein(a) and cholesteryl ester transfer. *Am. J. Clin. Nutr.* 77(5), 1119–1124.

[25] Mensink, R.P., Katan, M.B., (1990). Effect of dietary trans fatty acids on high-density and low-density lipoprotein cholesterol levels in healthy subjects. *N. Engl. J. Med.* 323, 439–445.

[26] Ascherio, A., Katan, M.B., Zock, P.L., Stampfer, M.J., Willett, W.C., (1999). Trans fatty acids and coronary heart disease. *N. Engl. J. Med.* 340(25), 1994–1998.

[27] Mensink, R.P., Zock, P.L., Kester, A.D., Katan, M.B., (2003). Effects of dietary fatty acids and carbohydrates on the ratio of serum total to HDL cholesterol and on serum lipids and apolipoproteins: a meta-analysis of 60 controlled trials. *Am. J. Clin. Nutr.* 77(5), 1146-55.

[28] Koletzko, B., Decsi, T., (1997). Metabolic aspects of trans fatty acids. *Clin. Nutr.* 16(5), 229–37.

[29] Brouwer, I.A., Wanders, A.J., Katan, M.B., (2010). Reitsma, Pieter H, ed. Effect of Animal and Industrial Trans Fatty Acids on HDL and LDL Cholesterol Levels in Humans – A Quantitative Review. *PLoS ONE* 5(3), e9434.

[30] Lopez-Garcia, E., Schulze, M.B., Meigs, J.B., Manson, J.E., Rifai, N., Stampfer, M.J., Willett, W.C., Hu, F.B., (2005). Consumption of Trans Fatty Acids Is Related to Plasma Biomarkers of Inflammation and Endothelial Dysfunction. *J. Nutr.* 135(3), 562–566.

[31] Mozaffarian, D., Rimm, E.B., King, I.B., Lawler, R.L., McDonald, G.B., Levy, W.C., (2004). Trans fatty acids and systemic inflammation in heart failure. *Am. J. Clin. Nutr.* 80, 1521-5.

[32] Mozaffarian, D., Pischon, T., Hankinson, S.E., Rifai, N., Joshipura, K., Willett, W.C., Rimm, E.B., (2004). Dietary intake of trans fatty ac-ids and systemic inflammation in women. *Am. J. Clin. Nutr.* 79, 606-12.

[33] Han, S.N., Leka, L.S., Lichtenstein, A.H., Ausman, L.M., Schaefer, E.J., Meydani, S.N., (2002). Ef-fect of hydrogenated and saturated, relative to polyunsaturated, fat on immune and inflammatory responses of adults with moderate hypercholesterolemia. *J. Lipid Res.* 43, 445-52.

[34] Baer, D.J., Judd, J.T., Clevidence, B.A., Tracy, R.P., (2004). Dietary fatty acids affect plasma markers of inflammation in healthy men fed controlled diets: a randomized crossover study. *Am. J. Clin. Nutr.* 79, 969-73.

[35] Vasan, R.S., Sullivan, L.M., Roubenoff, R., Dinarello, C.A., Harris, T., Benjamin, E.J., Sawyer, D.B., Levy, D., Wilson, P.W., D'Agostino, R.B., (2003). Inflammatory markers and risk of heart failure in elderly subjects without prior myocardial infarction: the Framing-ham Heart Study. *Circulation* 107, 1486-91.

[36] Pickup, J.C., (2004). Inflammation and activated innate immunity in the pathogenesis of type 2 diabetes. *Diabetes Care* 27, 813-23.

[37] Albert, C.M., Ma, J., Rifai, N., Stampfer, M.J., Ridker, P.M., (2002). Prospective study of C-reactive protein, homocysteine, and plasma lipid levels as predictors of sudden cardiac death. *Circulation* 105, 2595-9.

[38] Libby, P., Ridker, P.M., Maseri, A., (2002). Inflammation and atherosclerosis. *Circulation* 105, 1135-43.

[39] Ridker, P.M., Hennekens, C.H., Buring, J.E., Rifai, N., (2000). C-reactive protein and other markers of inflammation in the prediction of cardiovascular disease in women. *N. Engl. J. Med.* 342, 836-43.

[40] de Roos, N.M., Bots, M.L., Katan, M.B., (2001). Replacement of dietary saturated fatty acids by trans fatty acids lowers serum HDL cholesterol and impairs endothelial function in healthy men and women. *Arterioscler. Thromb. Vasc. Biol.* 21, 1233-7.

[41] Iwata, N.G., Pham, M., Rizzo, N.O., Cheng, A.M., Maloney, E., Kim, F., (2011). Trans Fatty Acids Induce Vascular Inflammation and Reduce Vascular Nitric Oxide Production in Endothelial Cells. *PLoS ONE* 6(12), e29600.

[42] Thomas, L.H., Winter, J.A., Scott, R.G., (1983). Concentration of trans unsaturated fatty acids in the adipose body tissue of decedents dying of ischaemic heart disease compared with controls. *J. Epidemiol. Community Health* 37, 22–24.

[43] Lemaitre, R.N., King, I.B., Raghunathan, T.E., Pearce, R.M., Weinmann, S., Knopp, R.H., Copass, M.K., Cobb, L.A., Siscovick, D.*S*., (2002). Cell membrane trans fatty acids and the risk of primary cardiac arrest. *Circulation* 105, 697–701.

[44] Dietary Guidelines Advisory Committee (DGAC), Nutrition and your health: dietary guidelines for Americans: 2005 Dietary Guidelines Advisory Committee report. Washington, D.C.: Department of Agriculture; 2005.

[45] Clifton, P.M., Keogh, J.B., Noakes, M., (2004). Trans fatty acids in adipose tissue and the food supply are associated with myocardial infarction. *J. Nutr. (Amer Inst Nutrition)* 134(4), 874–879.

[46] Stender, S., Dyerberg, J., Bysted, A., Leth, T., Astrup, A., (2006). A *trans* world journey. *Atheroscler. Suppl. (Elsevier)* 7(2), 47–52.

[47] Stender, S., Dyerberg, J., (2004). Influence of trans fatty acids on health. *Ann. Nutr. Metab.* 48(2), 61–6.

[48] Mozaffarian, D., Stampfer, M.J., (2010). Removing industrial *trans* fat from foods: A simple policy that will save lives. *BMJ.* 340, c1826.

[49] National Institute for Health and Clinical Excellence, Recommendations, *NICE public health guidance 25: Prevention of cardiovascular disease*. UK: Manchester; 2010. Retrieved 2013-03-12

[50] Food and nutrition board, institute of medicine of the national academies, *Dietary reference intakes for energy, carbohydrate, fiber, fat, fatty acids, cholesterol, protein, and amino acids (macronutrients)*. National Academies Press; 2005.

[51] National Dairy Council), Comments on 'Docket No. 2003N-0076 Food Labeling: Trans Fatty Acids in Nutrition Labeling' (PDF); 2004-06-18. Retrieved 2007-01-07.

[52] Tricon, S., Burdge, G.C., Kew, S., Banerjee, T., Russell, J.J., Jones, E.L., Grimble, R.F., Williams, C.M., Yaqoob, P., Calder, P.C., (2004). Opposing effects of cis-9,trans-11 and trans-10,cis-12 conjugated linoleic acid on blood lipids in most healthy humans. *Am. J. Clin. Nutr.* 80(3), 614–20.

[53] Zulet, M.A., Marti, A., Parra, M.D., Martínez, J.A., (2005). Inflammation and conjugated linoleic acid: mechanisms of action and implications for human health. *J. Physiol. Biochem.* 61(3), 483–94.

[54] Clarke, R., Lewington, S., (2006). Trans fatty acids and coronary heart disease: Food labels should list these as well as cholesterol and saturated fat. *Brit. Med. J.* 333(7561), 214.

Chapter 5

Over Consumption of Homocysteine-Increasing Diets

Homocysteine is an amino acid that contains sulfur and is not involved in comprising proteins. Its structure diagram is shown in Figure 10.

The homocysteine in the blood normally originates from two ways. One is that homocysteine is synthesized during the metabolism of methionine that is an essential amino acid and involved in comprising proteins. Methionine adenosyltransferase (an enzyme) catalyzes the conversion of methionine into S-adenosylmethionine. When the methyl group is donated to its acceptors (e.g. proteins, DNAs), S-adenosylmethionine is converted to S-adenosylhomocysteine. Then, homocysteine is produced when the adenosine of S-adenosylhomocysteine is removed by the catalysis of S-adenosylhomocysteine hydrolase. (This enzymatic reaction is reversible). Once formed, homocyateine biochemically plays a juncturral role that is critical in the metabolism of methionine and the bioproduction of cysteine (an amino acid comprising proteins) and taurine. Two biochemical pathways are normally involved in the metabolism of homocysteine. They are named re-methylation and trans-sulfuration. Re-methylation is necessary for the conversion of homocysteine back into methionine while trans-sulfuration is necessary for converting homocysteine to taurine and cysteine. When this biochemical process is impaired or broken down, an abnormally high concentration of homocysteine in the blood (or named hyperhomocysteinemia) can be detected. Another is that an increase in the intake of homocysteine included in diets or foods would elevate the level of homocysteine in the blood [1]. It should be noted that the level of serum homocysteine may be affected by genetic factors [2] and its content in the daily diet [1].

All those described in the above paragraphs mean that the level of homocysteine in the blood and the factors that affects its concentration in the blood should be very likely associated with human health. Because there are two mechanisms of elevating blood homocysteine, it becomes complicated when analyzing its connection with human health. Is the elevation of homocysteine in the blood is a causality of some adverse biochemical consequences or just an outcome of other impaired biochemical or physiological reactions? If it is just the outcome of other impaired biochemical or physiological reactions, does the dietary intake of homocysteine affect human health? Here in the following parts of this chapter, the association of dietary homocysteine with CVDs will be discussed.

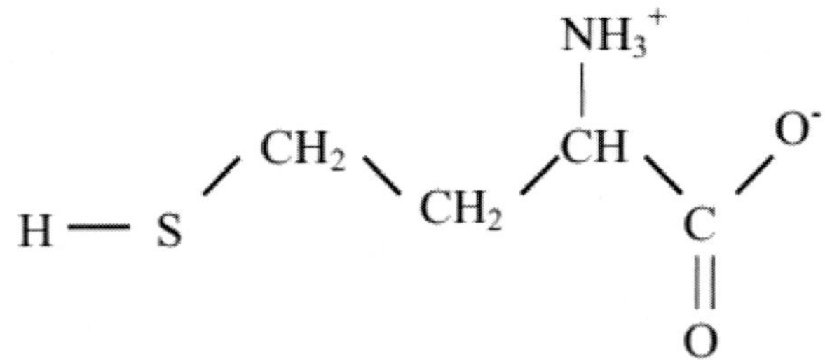

Figure 10. Structure diagram of homocysteine.

Homocysteine and CVDs

The normal basal level of homocysteine in healthy humans ranges from 5 to 15 μM, with an average concentration of 10 μM [3]. Hyperhomocysteinemia is defined as a serum homocysteine level >15 μmol/L [4]. It was also stated that between 16 and 30 μM, 31 and 100 μM and >100 μM are considered to be moderate, intermediate and severe hyperhomocysteinaemia, respectively [3].

There is a scientific consensus of believing that an increased homocysteine in the blood (hyperhomocysteinemia) is a reliable independent predictor of CVDs [5,6]. Furthermore, this conclusion about the positive association of hyperhomocysteinemia with CVDs has been supported by more scientific evidences [7]. It was also reported that an increase of 5 μmol/L in plasma would result in a 60% and 80% increase in the risk of CVDs in men and women, respectively [8]. Moreover, several investigations found that mild to moderate hyperhomocysteinemia was positively associated with macrovascular occlusion that is closely linked to peripheral, cerebrovascular and coronary atherosclerosis as well as venous thromboembolism [9]. It has also been concluded that the hyperhomocysteinemia is associated with microvasculopathy, especially diseases in cerebral small vessels [10]. The homocysteine with its concentration higher than 12 μM in plasma was found to be capable of elevating the risk of inducing the dysfunction of small vessels and the atherothrombosis of large vessels in individuals [11].

It seems that the mechanism for the positive association of the hyperhomocysteinemia with CVDs needs more studies to draw a conclusion. However, there are scientific evidences that are helpful for understanding the mechanism.

The toxicity of the hyperhomocysteinemia to blood vessels or heart muscles may be involved in the mechanism since it has been found to induce endothelial dysfunction, elevate thrombin formation, reduce native thrombolysis, increase lipid peroxidation, and promote vascular smooth muscle proliferation and monocyte chemotaxis [12-15]. The association of endothelial dysfunction with CVDs has been well described previously in "Chapter 2 Cholesterol".

The effect of promoting lipid peroxidation by homocysteines results from the formation of free radicals. There are several reports in the literature that stated the positive association of homocysteine with oxidative stress causing lipid peroxidation [16-20]. An increase in the level of homosysteine could cause oxidative stress that might adversely influence lipoprotein particles and subsequently impair endothelial cells [21]. Homocysteines are able to increase hydroxyl radical production of homocysteinylated- [22], nitrated- [23], or oxidized-LDL [21].

As compared to the native LDL particles, the LDL particles that are modified become more harmful because macrophages readily take them up and this process promotes the beginning and the further development of response of the inflammation in the endothelial lesions. Study on ApoE/mice indicated that the treatment of homocysteine elevated LDL particles that were oxidized [21]. The oxidation process may promote the amount of LDL particles taken up by scavenger receptors on macrophages or monocytes or in the aortic lesions so that the development of atherosclerosis is promoted. Furthermore, the elevation of reactive oxygen species caused by hyperhomocysteinemia is capable of stimulating the molecules of the signal transduction so that endothelial dysfunction is induced [24]. There are some scientific results that indicate the involvement of endothelial nitric oxide synthase in the pro-oxidant properties of homocysteine [25]. This may be proved by the fact that the level of plasma homocysteine can be decreased and that the oxidation of LDL and VLDL particles can be prevented by the supplementation of folate, obtained by carrying out an *in vivo* study [26]. There is a report in the literature which stated that lipid peroxidation was induced by the dietary supplementation of DL-homocysteines [27]. The authors found that the level of thiobarbituric acid reactive substances (a measure of lipid peroxidation) in heart tissues was significantly elevated by fed Sprague-Dawley rats with the diets containing 10 g/kg DL-homocysteines.

In addition, one report concluded that the homocysteine can interact with the "tail" domain of annexin 2 complex via a disulfide bond and therefore inhibits the annexin 2 complex-mediated activation (which is dependent upon Tissue Plasminogen Activator) of plasminogen *in vitro* [11]. The same authors also concluded that the derivatization of annexin 2 complex resulted in the impairment of fibrinolysis and postnatal angiogenesis since annexin 2 complex-deficient mice developed the impairment of fibrinolysis and postnatal angiogenesis. They ultimately concluded that the hyperhomocysteinemia caused the impairment of postnatal angiogenesis, the inhibition of directed endothelial cell migration and the prevention of perivascular fibrinolysis.

An increase in (micro)albumin caused by homocysteines may be another factor involving in the adverse effect on the cardiovascular system. It was found that the concentrations of homocysteine higher than 19 mmol/L at baseline significantly promoted the development of (micro)albuminuria, as compared to those concentrations lower than 9.1 mmol/L, which was analyzed by logistic regression [28]. The authors also stated that this result was obtained after the adjustment of glucose tolerance, sex and age while the result was not materially changed after an additional adjustment of estimates of glomerular filtration rate, current smoking, retinopathy, the presence of CVDs, body mass index, blood pressure and baseline insulin resistance. They also carried out an experiment which indicated the positive association of an elevated risk of developing (micro)albuminuria with a 5 mmol/L elevation of the homocysteine concentration. Microalbuminuria refers to the urinary excretion of albumin that is slightly increased, as compared to the normal (or healthy) condition. It was found that the microalbuminuria is positively linked to an elevated risk of mortality and morbidity of CVDs in individuals with nondiabetic diseases or non–insulin-dependent diabetes mellitus [29,30].

The adverse effect of homocysteines on lipid profile may also be one of the factors involved in increasing the risk of CVDs. An experimental study indicated that the increased level of homocyateines in the blood was able to decrease HDLC concentration [31]. The authors also concluded that the decrease in HDLC resulted from the inhibition of production of the main HDL apolipoprotein (ApoA) -I without the reduction of ApoA-I mRNA, in the liver. This conclusion related to the inhibition of ApoA-I production by homocysteines was supported by another study [32]. This investigation also found that the synthesis of ApoA-I was decreased by homocysteines though the authors stated a different cause (i.e. the reduction of ApoA-I mRNA) from the former reported study. The authors stated that homocysteines may reduce the expression of ApoA-I via decreasing peroxisome proliferator receptor alpha (the transcription factor), which involves in ApoA-I transcription [32]. The only fly in the ointment is that it seems difficult to find reports in the past literature investigating into other lipid particles, such as LDLC, TC, since the HDLC/LDLC or TC ratio is a more powerful predictor of CVDs than each of them alone (see Chapter 1 and 2 discussed above in this book).

The enhancing effect of homocysteine on the adhesion between endothelial cells and neutrophils may be another factor for increasing the risk of CVDs. For example, it was indicated that the presence of homocysteine resulted in purified human peripheral blood neutrophils binding to human umbilical vein endothelial cells, with dose-response curves that are almost identical [33]. It was also reported that the increases in homocysteine concentrations from ≤10 mmol/L to ≥200 mmol/L progressively elevated neutrophil adhesion by about 50% [34]. The same authors also stated that homocysteines at pathophysiological concentrations *in vitro* resulted in the elevated adhesion between endothelial cells and neutrophils, and the contact can cause the migration of neutrophils across the endothelial layer, inducing the detachment and concurrent damage of endothelial cells. The elevated adhesion was associated with changes in the surface of the neutrophils, but no alteration of the endothelial surface adhesion molecules (i.e. VCAM-1, E-selectin, ICAM-1) [33] and P-selectin was detected [34].

Controversial views also exist: more studies needed to conclude that moderately elevated homocysteines result in CVDs, though the level of serum homocysteines is a powerful prognostic marker of mortality and CVD events in patients with preexisting CVD risk factors [35]. Furthermore, it was reported that the hyperhomocysteinemia induced by a methionine-enriched diet did not cause an adverse effect on the level of plasma lipids [36]. Although it is not found that the association of an elevated homocysteine concentration in the blood with an elevated risk of CVDs in individuals can be proved by all observational epidemiological studies, it can be ratified by most of these studies. About 80% of retrospective case-control investigations and 20% of prospective investigations indicate a positive association of an elevated homocysteine concentration in the blood with an elevated risk of CVDs in individuals [9]. The study on the effect of homocysteine supplementations in drinking water (0.9-1.8 g/L) also observed the acceleration of aortic plaque [37].

Dietary Sources of Increasing Blood Homocysteine

According to all the contexts described in the above paragraphs or sections, it might be reasonable in believing that the dietary sources of increasing blood homocysteines should not be ignored for the prevention of CVDs. Although the number of the literature presently available is very limited, there are some reports relating to diets, the level of blood homocysteine, and CVDs.

The significant dietary sources of increasing the level of blood homocysteines might be mainly methionine-rich foods or diets. For example, it was indicated that young ApoE-deficient mice fed the diet (enriched with methionine (7.7 g/kg diet) combined B vitamins deficiency) for 56 days developed severe hyperhomocysteinemia [38]. (The association of B vitamins with CVDs has been discussed in detail in Chapter 3 Malnutrition.) These authors also observed 2 times increases in the size of aortic plaque and the increased complexity of lesions. Another study found that the food supplemented with methionine (22–44 g/kg diet) induced the hyperhomocysteinemia and the accelerated aortic plaque [37]. It should also be noted that the association of homocysteines with CVDs might be underlain by some outcomes of excessive methionine metabolism rather than increased blood homocysteines per se [39].

The consumption of proteins is a significant source of influencing the level of blood homocysteine. The most important factors for increasing the level of blood homocysteines are the origin and amount of the proteins consumed. For example, it was found that the increased consumption of the diet rich in animal-proteins elevated the level of blood homocysteine whereas the increased consumption of the high plant-protein diet decreased the concentration of blood homocysteines [40]. The same authors also stated that the total amount of proteins ingested was greatly associated with the total levels of blood homocysteines. Another study also found a positive association of an increased animal protein intake with an increase in blood homocysteines [41]. The possible reason for this observed result is the increased consumption of eggs, organ meats, dairy products, milk, chicken and red meats that contain large amounts of methionine [42].

The increased consumption of SFAs is also positively associated with the elevation of the total plasma homocysteine level. For example, it was reported that the level of homocysteine in the blood was increased by increasing dietary SFA ingestion [43]. This study ultimately included 5917 persons divided into 2 groups according to age (i.e. 47–49 and 71–74 years old) and the amount of SFAs consumed was obtained by the calculation according to the food intake and composition tables. This conclusion may be indirectly supported by the study found that the blood homocysteine level was down-regulated by increasing the consumption of polyunsaturated fatty acids [44].

Alcoholism can also induce the hyperhomocysteinemia (see "Chapter 3 Malnutrition" for the association of alcohol with CVDs). It was reported that alcoholics who hospitalized for detoxification had an elevated level of homocysteines in the blood, as compared to controls [45]. The authors also noted that the level of blood homocysteine in abstinent alcoholics was not different from that of controls. They assumed that the elevated level of blood homocysteine in alcoholics might be responsible for the elevated morbidity of strokes observed in these individuals. Another study suggested that the mechanism of increasing the level of homocysteine in the blood by the chronic ingestion of alcohol should involve the interference of methionine synthase activity [46]. The authors found that chronic alcoholics had the blood homocysteine level 2 times higher than that in nondrinkers, the significant lower level of folate in red blood cells and pyridoxal 5'-phosphate in serum than that controls did whereas the significant lower levels of homocysteine were found in beer drinkers than that in wine or spirits drinkers.

The consumption of coffee could also increase the concentration of blood homocysteine. For example, a study involved 8585 women and 7589 men aged 40-67 years old indicated a significant positive dose-response relationship between the level of total homocysteine in plasma and the consumption of coffee, which was stronger than that between TC in serum and the consumption of ccffee [47]. These authors found that the drinkers of 9 cups of coffee/day had 12.0 μmol/L of the average total homocysteine in the blood in 40-42 years old men whereas nonusers had 10.1 μmol/L. Correspondingly, 10.5 and 8.2 μmol/L of the average total homocysteine were respectively found in 40-42 years old women. They also stated that after the adjustment for the lower ingestion of vitamin supplements or fruits or vegetables and smoking, the correlation between the consumption of coffee and the total level of homocysteine in the blood was varied only moderately. They further concluded that if the high ingestion of coffee combined with cigarette smoking, the particularly high levels of the total homocysteine in the blood were detected. They also concluded that tea drinking was negatively associated with the total level of homocysteine in the blood after the adjustment of coffee drinking and smoking were undertaken. Another study also concluded that the consumption of coffee increased the total level of homocysteine in the blood [48]. The results of this study resulted from a randomized crossover trial involved 64 Dutch women and men. In this experiment, half of the subjects drank 1 L unfiltered coffee/day for 14 days and another half drank broth, tea, chocolate drink, milk, or water for 14 days. After the washout was undertaken for 56 days, they repeated the experiment and switched the treatments. At the end of each treatment period, they sampled blood.

It seems that the contribution of dietary homocysteine sources to the hyperhomocysteinemia is quite limited. The homocysteine exists in many food resources such as tuna, swine liver, Roquefort cheese, beer, and white bread [13]. The significance of the homocysteine in these foods in term of contributing to the level of homocysteine in the blood needs further studies to make a conclusion since the animal products among them should also contain abundant amounts of methionine (see second and third paragraphs in this section). The level of homocysteine in red wine or white wine was found to be 10.31±4.25 μM or 6.11±3.44 μM, respectively [49]. Although its content in vegetables is quite low, it is very ample in sprouted alfalfa or beans seeds (sprouted soy beans commonly eaten as a vegetable in China) [50]. The authors measured the homocysteine content in 58 food items and concluded that their contribution to the level of blood homocysteine should be nonsignificant. However, if the concentration of homocysteine in foods or diets is high, their effects of increasing the level of blood homocysteine may not be ignorable. For example, it was reported that the supplementation of homocysteine in drinking water (0.9–1.8 g/L) significantly increased the level of blood homocysteine and accelerated aortic plaque [36].

References

[1] Pexa, A., Fischer, K., Deussen, A., Henle, T., (2008). Homocysteine in food. *Eur. Food Res. Technol.* 226(4), 933-935.

[2] Qin, X., Li, J., Cui, Y., Liu, Z., Zhao, Z., Ge, J., Guan, D., Hu, J., Wang, Y., Zhang, F., Xu, X., Wang, X., Xu, X., Huo. Y., (2012). MTHFR C677T and MTR A2756G polymorphisms and the homocysteine lowering efficacy of different doses of folic acid in hypertensive Chinese adults. *Nutr. J.* 11, 2-8.

[3] Stopper, H., Treutlein1, A.T., Bahner, U., Schupp, N., Schmid, U., Brink, A., Perna, A., Heidland, A., (2008). Reduction of the genomic damage level in haemodialysis patients

by folic acid and vitamin B12 supplementation. *Nephrol. Dial. Transplant.* 23, 3272–3279.

[4] Jacques, P.F., Selhub, J., Bostom, A.G., Wilson, P.W., Rosenberg, I.H., (1999). The effect of folic acid fortification on plasma folate and total homocysteine concentrations. *N. Engl. J. Med.* 340, 1449–54.

[5] Wilcken, D.E., Wilcken, B., (1976). The pathogenesis of coronary artery disease. A possible role for methionine metabolism. *J. Clin. Invest.* 57, 1079–1082.

[6] Refsum, H., Ueland, P.M., Nygard, O., Vollset, S.E., (1998). Homocysteine and cardiovascular disease. *Annu. Rev. Med.* 49, 31–62.

[7] Debreceni, B., Debreceni, L., (2014). The role of homocysteine-lowering B-vitamins in the primary prevention of cardiovascular disease. *Cardiovasc. Ther.* 32(3), 130-8.

[8] Boushey, C.J., Beresford, S.A.A., Omenn, G.S., Motulsky, A.G., (1995). A quantitative assessment of plasma homocysteine as a risk factor for vascular disease. Probable benefits of increasing folic acid intakes. *J. Am. Med. Assoc.* 274, 1049–57.

[9] Nygard, O., Nordrehaug, J.E., Refsum, H., Ueland, P.M., Farstad, M., Vollset, S.E., (1997). Plasma homocysteine levels and mortality in patients with coronary artery disease. *N. Engl. J. Med.* 337, 230–236.

[10] Markus, H.S., (2007). Genes, endothelial function and cerebral small vessel disease in man. *Exp. Physiol.* 93, 121–127.

[11] Jacovina, A.T., Deora, A.B., Ling, Q., Broekman, M.J., Almeida, D., Greenberg, C.B., Marcus, A.J., Smith, J.D., Hajjar, K.A., (2009). Homocysteine inhibits neoangiogenesis in mice through blockade of annexin A2–dependent fibrinolysis. *J. Clin. Invest.* 119, 3384–3394

[12] Splaver, A., Lamas, G.A., Hennekens, C.H., (2004). Homocysteine and cardiovascular disease: biological mechanisms, observational epidemiology, and the need for randomized trials. *Am. Heart J.* 148, 34–40.

[13] Jacobsen, D.W., Catanescu, O., Dibello, P.M., Barbato, J.C., (2005). Molecular targeting by homocysteine: a mechanism for vascular pathogenesis. *Clin. Chem. Lab. Med.* 43, 1076–83.

[14] Moat, S.J., McDowell, I.F., (2005). Homocysteine and endothelial function in human studies. *Semin. Vasc. Med.* 5, 172–182.

[15] Wilson, K.M., Lentz, S.R., (2005). Mechanisms of the atherogenic effects of elevated homocysteine in experimental models. *Semin. Vasc. Med.* 5, 163–171.

[16] Coppola, A., Davi, G., de Stefano, V., Mancini, F.P., Cerbone, A.M., di Minno, G., (2000). Homocysteine, coagulation, platelet function and thrombosis. *Semin. Thromb. Hemost.* 26, 243-254.

[17] Perna, A.F., Ingrosso, D., de Santo, N.G., (2003). Homocysteine and oxidative stress. *Amino Acids* 25, 409-417.

[18] Weiss, N., (2005). Mechanisms of increased vascular oxidant stress in hyperhomocysteinemia and its impact on endothelial function. *Curr. Drug Metab.* 6, 27-36.

[19] Castelao, J.E., Gago-Dominguez, M., (2008). Risk factors for cardiovascular disease in women: Relationship to lipid peroxidation and oxidative stress. *Med. Hypotheses* 71, 39-44.

[20] Khosrowbeygi, A., Lorzadeh, N., Ahmadvand, H., Shiravand, Y., (2011). Homocysteine and its Association with Lipid Peroxidation and Leptin in Preeclampsia. *Intern. J. Biol. Chem.* 5(3), 184-192.

[21] Thampi, P., Stewart, B.W., Joseph, L., Melnyk, S.B., Hennings, L.J., Nagarajan, S., (2008). Dietary homocysteine promotes atherosclerosis in apoE-deficient mice by inducing scavenger receptors expression. *Atheroscler.* 197, 620–629.

[22] Ferretti, G., Bacchetti, T., Moroni, C., Vignini, A., Nanetti, L., Curatola, G., (2004). Effect of homocysteinylation of low density lipoproteins on lipid peroxidation of human endothelial cells. *J. Cell. Biochem.* 92, 351–360.

[23] Griffiths, H.R., Aldred, S., Dale, C., Nakano, E., Kitas, G.D., Grant, M.G., Nugent, D., Taiwo, F.A., Li, L., Powers, H.J., (2006). Homocysteine from endothelial cells promotes LDL nitration and scavenger receptor uptake. *Free Radic. Biol. Med.* 40, 488–500.

[24] Foncea, R., Carvajal, C., Almarza, C., Leighton, F., (2000). Endothelial cell oxidative stress and signal transduction. *Biol. Res.* 33, 89–96.

[25] Heydrick, S.J., Weiss, N., Thomas, S.R., Cap, A.P., Pimentel, D.R., Loscalzo, J., Keaney, J.F., (2004). L-Homocysteine and L-homocystine stereospecifically induce endothelial nitric oxide synthase-dependent lipid peroxidation in endothelial cells. *Free Radic. Biol. Med.* 36, 632–640.

[26] McEneny, J., Couston, C., McKibben, B., Young, I.S., Woodside, J.V., (2007). Folate: in vitro and in vivo effects on VLDL and LDL oxidation. *Int. J. Vitam. Nutr. Res.* 77, 66–72.

[27] Brown, O.W., Strain, J.J., (1990). Effect of Dietary Homocysteine on Copper Status in Rats. *J. Nutr.* 120, 1068-1074.

[28] Jager, A., Kostense, P.J., Nijpels, G., Dekker, J.M., Heine, R.J., Bouter, L.M., Donker, A.J.M., Stehouwer, C.D.A., (2001). Serum Homocysteine Levels Are Associated With the Development of (Micro)albuminuria (The Hoorn Study). *Arterioscler. Thromb. Vasc. Biol.* 21, 74-81.

[29] Dinneen, S.F., Gerstein, H.C., (1997). The association of microalbuminuria and mortality in non-insulin-dependent diabetes mellitus: a systematic overview of the literature. *Arch. Intern. Med.* 157, 1413–1418.

[30] Yudkin, J.S., Forrest, R.D., Jackson, C.A., (1988). Microalbuminuria as predictor of vascular disease in non-diabetic subjects: Islington Diabetes Survey. *Lancet.* 2, 530 – 533.

[31] Liao, D., Tan, H., Hui, R., Li, Z., Jiang, X., Gaubatz, J., Yang, F., Durante, W., Chan, L., Schafer, A.I., Pownall, H.J., Yang, X., Wang, H., (2006). Hyperhomocysteinemia decreases circulating HDL by inhibiting apoA-I protein synthesis and enhancing HDL-C clearance. *Circ. Res.* 99, 598–606.

[32] Mikael, L.G., Genest, J., Rozen, R., (2006). Elevated homocysteine reduces apolipoprotein A-I expression in hyperhomocysteinemic mice and in males with coronary artery disease. *Circ. Res.* 98, 564–571.

[33] Dudman, N.P.B., Hale, S.E.T., Endothelial- and leukocyte-mediated mechanisms in homocysteine-associated occlusive vascular disease. In: Graham I, Refsum H, Rosenberg IH, Ueland PM, eds. Homocysteine Metabolism: From Basic Science to Clinical Medicine. Boston, Mass: Kluwer Academic; 1997; pp.267–271.

[34] Dudman, N.P.B., Temple, S.E., Guo, X.W., Fu, W., Perry, M.A., (1999). Homocysteine Enhances Neutrophil-Endothelial Interactions in Both Cultured Human Cells and Rats In Vivo. *Circ. Res.* 84, 409-416.

[35] Refsum, H., Nurk, E., Smith, A.D., Ueland, P.M., Gjesdal, C.G., Bjelland, I., Tverdal, A., Tell, G.S., Nygård, O., Vollset, S.E., (2006). The Hordaland homocysteine study: A community-based study of homocysteine, its determinants, and associations with disease. *J. Nutr.* 136, 1731S–1740S.

[36] Zhou, J., Werstuck, G.H., Lhotak, S., Shi, Y.Y., Tedesco, V., Trigatti, B., Dickhout, J., Majors, A.K., DiBello, P.M., Jacobsen, D.W., Austin, R.C., (2008). Hyperhomocysteinemia induced by methionine supplementation does not independently cause atherosclerosis in C57BL/6J mice. *FASEB J.* 22, 2569– 2578.

[37] Zhou, J., Moller, J., Danielsen, C. C., Bentzon, J., Ravn, H. B., Austin, R. C., Falk, E., (2001). Arterioscler. *Thromb. Vasc. Biol.* 21, 1470–1476.

[38] Hofmann, M. A., Lalla, E., Lu, Y., Gleason, M. R., Wolf, B. M., Tanji, N., Ferran, L. J., Jr., Kohl, B., Rao, V., Kisiel, W., Stern, D.M., Schmidt, A.M., (2001). Hyperhomocysteinemia enhances vascular inflammation and accelerates atherosclerosis in a murine model. *J. Clin. Invest.* 107, 675–683.

[39] Troen, A.M., Lutgens, E., Smith, D.E., Rosenberg, I.H., Selhub, J., (2003). The atherogenic effect of excess methionine intake. *PNAS.* 100(25), 15089–15094.

[40] Xiao, X., Zhang, Y., Wang, M., Li, X., Xia, M., Ling, W., (2013). Dietary protein and plasma total homocysteine, cysteine concentrations in coronary angiographic subjects. *Nutr. J.* 12, 144.

[41] Yakub, M., Iqbal, M.P., Iqbal, R., (2010). Dietary patterns are associated with hyperhomocysteinemia in an urban Pakistani population. *J. Nutr.* 140(7), 261–1266.

[42] Tucker, K.L., Selhub, J., Wilson, P.W., Rosenberg, I.H., (1996). Dietary intake pattern relates to plasma folate and homocysteine concentrations in the Framingham Heart Study. *J. Nutr.* 126(12), 3025–3031.

[43] Berstad, P., Konstantinova, S.V., Refsum, H., Nurk, E., Vollset, S.E., Tell, G.S., Ueland, P.M., Drevon, C.A., Ursin, G., (2007). Dietary fat and plasma total homocysteine concentrations in 2 adult age groups: the Hordaland Homocysteine Study. *Am. J. Clin. Nutr.* 85(6), 1598–1605.

[44] Huang, T., Tucker, K.L., Lee, Y.C., Crott, J.W., Parnell, L.D., Shen, J., Smith, C.E., Ordovas, J.M., Li, D., Lai, C.Q., (2011). Methylenetetrahydrofolate reductase variants associated with hypertension and cardiovascular disease interact with dietary polyunsaturated fatty acids to modulate plasma homocysteine in puerto rican adults. *J. Nutr.* 141(4), 654–659.

[45] Hultberg, B., Berglund, M., Andersson, A., Frank, A., (1993). Elevated plasma homocysteine in alcoholics. *Alcohol Clin. Exp. Res.* 17(3), 687–689.

[46] Cravo, M.L., Gloria, L.M., Selhub, J., Nadeau, M.R., Camilo, M.E., Resende, M.P., Cardoso, J.N., Leitão, C.N., Mira, F.C., (1996). Hyperhomocysteinemia in chronic alcoholism: correlation with folate, vitamin B-12, and vitamin B-6 status. *Am. J. Clin. Nutr.* 63, 220-224.

[47] Nygard, O., Refsum, H., Ueland, P.M., Stensvold, I., Nordrehaug, J.E., Kvåle, G., Vollset, S.E., (1997). Coffee consumption and plasma total ho-mocysteine: The Hordaland Homocysteine Study. *Am. J. Clin. Nutr.* 65, 136-143.

[48] Grubben, M.J., Boers, G.H., Blom, H.J., Broekhuizen, R., de Jong, R., van Rijt, L., de Ruijter, E., Swinkels, D.W., Nagengast, F.M., Katan, M.B., (2000). Unfiltered coffee increases plasma homocysteine concentrations in healthy volunteers: a randomized trial. *Am. J. Clin. Nutr.* 71, 480–4.

[49] Glowacki, R., Borowczyk, K. and Bald, E., (2012). Fast analysis of wine for total homocysteine content by high-performance liquid chromatography. *Amino Acids* 42, 247-251.

[50] Sakamoto, A., Nishimura, Y., Ono, H., Sakura, N., (2002). Betaine and homocysteine concentrations in foods. *Pediatr. Int.* 44(4), 409-13.

Chapter 6

Consumption of Soft Drinks

A soft drink may be defined as an artificially designed and produced beverage that contains less than 0.5% alcohol. Typically, this kind of drink is made of carbonated water and sweeteners (perhaps also including flavorings). The sweeteners may usually be sugars (e.g. sucrose, high-fructose corn syrup, glucose, fructose, maltose), and sugar substitutes (for making diet drinks) or the combination of some of these sweeteners. Sometimes, preservatives, colorings, caffeine, and other ingredients may also be included in a soft drink. However, such non-alcoholic drinks as natural mineral water, teas, coffee, cocoa, undiluted fruit or vegetable juices, protein drinks, and other non-alcoholic beverages that are principally different from the above definition may not be considered as soft drinks.

The actual composition of soft drinks may vary with the variation of ingredients employed in making them. The dietary safety of soft drinks sold in the market may also vary. It should not be wise to say that all soft drinks are not healthy. But, some ingredients that are usually included in soft drinks do have adverse effects on the cardiovascular system. If their use in soft drinks is not stopped, they should continuously risk the cardiovascular health of consumers. In 2014, China consumed about 167 million tons soft drinks, including about 18 million tons carbonated water. Although Japanese did not commonly drink soft drinks, they are widely available nowadays in Japan [1]. In USA, it was estimated that 9.2% of the total energy intake was contributed by sugar-sweetened soft drinks in 2001 [2]. In 2005, the average consumption of added sugar was 64 kg per person [3] while 1/3 total daily sugar ingestion was contributed by soft drinks [4,5]. The rate of soft drinks consumed by teenagers and children is usually high in the society [6,7]. Soft drinks are consumed world widely. Therefore, the effect of consumption of soft drinks on human health, especially on the cardiovascular system is attracting more and more attentions. The main purpose of this chapter is to discuss the association of consumption of soft drinks with CVDs.

Common Ingredients Increasing CVD Risks

Traditionally, sugars are the most common sweeteners that are widely employed in making soft drinks. Their content in soft drinks is typically 100–150 g/L [4]. The most abundant and used sugar is sucrose. It is a disaccharide consisting of one glucose molecule and one fructose molecule. Nowadays, high-fructose corn syrup has been widely employed in making beverages and other sweet foods. For example, sucrose has been substituted by the high-fructose corn syrup that has now become the main sweetener added to soft drinks in the United States [8]. The high-fructose corn syrup is produced by initially hydrolyzing starch into glucose and then converting the glucose to fructose via an isomerization process in an industrial scale. There are two kinds of high-fructose corn syrup. Both types consist of glucose and fructose. The difference is that one contains 42% fructose while another one contains 55% fructose. Because of cheap raw materials and the low cost processing technology, the production of the high-fructose corn syrup costs less than that of sucrose does. This might be the reason of the high-fructose corn syrup being an attractive selection as a major sweetener. The high-fructose corn syrup is mainly employed in making soft drinks though it is also used for sweetening other manufactured foods for example sweets, canned fruits, cakes, and even breads. Glucose may also be employed in making energetic soft drinks for sports men or women. About the positive association of these saccharides with CVDs has been well discussed in "Chapter 3 Malnutrition" of this book. However, once contained in soft drinks, these saccharides may behave differently in term of affecting the cardiovascular system, as compared to their presence in other foods. There are presently seven non-nutritive sweeteners or sugar substitutes (Luo han guo extract, stevia, neotame, acesulfame potassium, aspartame, saccharin, and sucralose) that are approved by the U.S. Food and Drug Administration and are widely employed in a lots of processed foods [9]. Luo han guo extract and stevia sweeteners are extracted from natural plant materials. Neotame, acesulfame potassium, aspartame, saccharin, and sucralose are artificially produced sweeteners. These sweeteners may also be used in some kinds of diet soft drinks. It seems that their effect on the human cardiovascular system has not been studied as extensively as that of sugars has. There is a study involved obese people who do not normally ingest non-nutritive sweeteners, which concluded that the glycemic and insulin responses to an oral glucose load were affected by sucralose [9]. There are reports that have listed the side effects of the artificial sweeteners, i.e. 2 mg/kg/day of neotame causing headache (having hepatotoxic toxicity at higher doses), lower birth rate and weight loss (due to the consumption at higher doses), 15 mg/kg/day of acesulfame potassium causing headache, clastogenic and genotoxic toxicity at high doses and throid tumors in rats, 50 mg/kg/day of aspartame causing headache, dry mouth, dizziness, mood change, nausea, vomiting, reduced seizure threshold, thrombocytopenia, lymphomas and leukemias in rats, 5 mg/kg/day of saccharin causing nausea, vomiting, diarrhea, cancer in the offspring of breast-fed animals, low birth weight, bladder cancer and hepatotoxicity, and 5 mg/kg/day of sucralose causing diarrhea, thymus shrinkage and cecal enlargements in rats [10,11]. Therefore, the application of the artificial sweeteners to industry is currently quite limited. However, there is a tendency of developing soft drinks for improving the cardiovascular health by using sugar substitutes (including artificial sweeteners).

Consumption of Soft Drinks and CVDs

There are some epidemiological studies in humans that investigated the chronic effect of high-sugar soft drinks on human health. They appear to indicate an adverse effect of sugar sweetened soft drinks on the cardiovascular system in humans.

A cohort study involving 84,085 females followed for 28 years (1980–2008) and 43,371 males followed for 22 years (1986–2008) indicated that sugar-sweetened soft drinks and low-calorie soft drinks were associated with a significantly higher risk of strokes [13]. The authors found 2938 strokes in females for a period of 2,188,230 person-years of follow-up and 1416 strokes in males for a period of 841,770 person-years of follow-up. They also stated that 1 serving of caffeinated coffee/day reduced 9% stroke risks and 1 serving of decaffeinated coffee/day reduced 10% risks, as compared to 1 serving of sugar-sweetened soda/day. Similarly, 1 serving of low-calorie soda resulted in a similar decrease in stroke risks, as compared to 1 serving of de-caffeinated or caffeinated coffee [13]. This study was carried out in the United States of America. The authors did not state what kind of the artificial sweetener was in the low-calorie soft drinks. And also, they did not compare other components or criteria of the sugar-sweetened soft drinks and low-calorie soft drinks in addition to sugars and artificial sweeteners. If the other components or criteria of both soft drinks are the same, the presence of sugars is likely to be responsible for rising the stroke risks.

There is another study found the positive association of sugar sweetened soft drinks with strokes. It is a prospective study carried in Japan. The subjects participated in the study involved 39,786 Japanese females and males who were 40–59 years old. The definition of the soft drinks investigated in the study was as the following: caloric sweeteners-containing non-alcoholic beverages. The caloric sweeteners were mainly sugars, for example, high-fructose corn syrup or sucrose. Non-100% fruit juices, flavored juices and cola-type beverages are the soft drinks investigated. The investigation did not involve 100% vegetable or fruit juices. The investigation was undertaken from 1990 to 2008. The results of the investigation indicated that the number of subjects with strokes was 1922 (including 1047 ischemic and 859 hemorrhagic strokes) and that with an ischemic heart disease was 453 for a period of 18 years follow-up. The authors concluded that there was a positive association of consumption of soft drinks with the increased risk of ischemic strokes for females [13]. They also concluded that there was an inverse association of consumption of soft drinks with the risks of ischemic and total strokes for males though it is not significant, and the inverse trend was weakened when participants with baseline comorbidities or early incident cases were excluded. And also, the association of the risk of ischemic heart diseases and or hemorrhagic strokes with the consumption of soft drinks was not found in either sex [13]. This study again indicates that the presence of sugars in soft drinks is likely to be responsible for increasing the risk of some strokes, e.g. ischemic strokes for females (not for males).

A study involved 6039 subjects (at the average age of 52.9 years; 3470 in women) indicated that the consumption of sugar sweetened soft drinks (carbonated soft drinks) might increase CVD risks [14]. The authors generally concluded that the consumption of more than one soft drink per day caused a 48% more morbidity of metabolic syndromes in middle-aged individuals, as compared to that of less than one soft drink daily. They defined the metabolic syndrome as 3 or more of the following criteria observed: HDLC $<$ 50 mg/dL (female) or 40 mg/dL (male); blood pressure $\geq$135/85 mm Hg; serum triglycerides $\geq$ 150 mg/dL; fasting blood glucose $\geq$ 100 mg/dL; waist circumference $\geq$ 40 inches (male) or $\geq$ 35 inches (female). The factors, including glycemic indexes, the dietary ingestion of total calories, magnesium, fibers, trans fats and saturated fats, smoking, physical activity, sex and age that may affect the criteria listed above were adjusted for. An average of 4 years follow-up observation indicated that the rate of new-onset metabolic syndromes in subjects who had $\geq$1 soft drink daily was 21.6% whereas that in those who had $<$1 soft drink daily was only 17.8%. The intake of $\geq$ 1 soft drink daily was associated with a low HDLC level, hypertriglyceridemia, a higher blood pressure, impaired fasting glucose, and an increased waist circumference and obesity.

A recent study showed the significant association of intake of sugar-sweetened drinks with increased plasma C-reactive proteins and triglycerides, and decreased adiponectins as well as the consumption of artificially sweetened drinks with a lower C-peptide level [15]. Because the authors did not state what the artificial sweetener was, this investigation could not tell whether sodium carbonate or the sweetener in the soda drink is the main risk factor of CVDs or not. However, it was reported that the consumption of sodium-rich carbonated mineral water reduced CVDs in postmenopausal women [16].

Caffeine is also commonly added to many kinds of soft drinks, the level of which usually ranges from approximately 10 to 15 mg/100 ml. Therefore, the second largest source of total caffeine consumption is soft drinks so that teenagers and children primarily ingest caffeine by drinking caffeinated soft drinks [17]. The level of caffeine in soft drinks is normally supposed to be much less than the dosages of acutely increasing blood pressure that have been indicated. However, an investigation involving 155,000 females appeared to indicate that the intake of caffeine that was included in soft drinks more likely induced hypertension, as compared to that in coffee [18]. Metabolic studies showed that when the similar doses of caffeine were consumed alone, they may not be high enough to excite thermogenesis which is able to enhance the thermogenic impacts of sympathetic excitation induced by other molecules [19]. However, when the doses of caffeine are included in soft drinks with the presence of sugars, they might cause health problems. For example, the autonomic responses of the human body to the intake of sugars might be potentially modified by caffeines, which may acutely impair the regulation of the cardiovascular system [4]. Literature search appears to show that the number of investigation into the association of caffeine added to soft drinks with an increased risk of CVDs is quite limited. Nevertheless, the coexistence of caffeine and sugars might be more harmful though further study is needed to prove this assumption. Furthermore, caffeines in soft drinks without the presence of sugars might also potentially have adverse effects on the cardiovascular system (see Chapter 7 Adverse Effects of Alkaloids).

Generally, people do not only have soft drinks alone. They frequently have soft drinks when they have a meal. Especially, people usually have large amounts of soft drinks when they eat a fast food in restaurants [20]. If they eat a very fatty meal together with large quantities of soft drinks, they should be more cautious of causing health problems. Normally, the intake of a highly fatty meal elevates the level of triglycerides in the blood, which would be able to cause endothelial dysfunction for a couple of hours since taking the meal [21]. The intake of a highly fatty meal together with a sugar (e.g. especially fructose)-sweetened soft drink or sugars is very likely to enlarge the postprandial elevation of triglycerides in plasma [22]. If the meal eaten is a fast food or meal which contains high content of sugars and fats, it would potentially further enhance postprandial endothelial dysfunction, probably resulting in an extra increase in CVD risks [4].

The acutely postprandial changes of physiological processes in the human body for a long term might be able to induce the development of CVDs [23]. Particularly, diets that contain large amounts of sugars and lipids are capable of resulting in an impaired 'postprandial metabolism', such as an elevated sympathetic activity, endothelial dysfunction and oxidative stress [24]. It appears that the association of intake of soft drinks with hypertension in humans has not yet been comprehensively studied though there are animal studies reported in the literature that illustrated the potential association of high-sugar meals with hypertension. However, it seems that there have been some studies on the effects of sugars in soft drinks on the cardiovascular system. Although acutely postprandial changes of physiological processes occasionally occurred may not cause a cardiovascular problem, this kind of acute effect repeated frequently enough might be able to result in cumulative harmful impacts. The acute impacts of fructose and glucose ingestion on the regional blood flow and sympathetic activity (also see Chapter 3 Malnutrition) were also estimated by investigations into the human body. For example, the effects of these monosaccharides on the vascular tone were reported to be importantly different [4] though both glucose and fructose were found to lead to the sympathetic activation of heart and subsequently elevate the heart rate [25-27]. Although the infusion of fructose did not increase the sympathetic activity of muscle nerves and result in vasodilatation in skeletal muscles, that of glucose did [28]. The hemodynamic action of insulin, which leads to vasodilatation in the skeletal muscles, might explain the opposite vascular responses to glucose and fructose [29]. The effect of acute intake of fructose on the secretion of insulin was found to be negligible, as compared to that of glucose [30,31]. The intake of fructose can increase the cardiac output and this accompanied by a lack of peripheral vasodilatation that is mediated by insulin would hence have the potential of acutely elevating blood pressure [4]. By recruiting volunteers who are healthy young, the acute effects of ingesting fructose and glucose were compared by carrying out a randomized crossover trial [32]. The authors reported that the intake of a 500 ml soft drink which contains 60 g fructose greatly elevated blood pressure for more than 2 h since the drink was taken. They also observed that the elevation of blood pressure which was caused by the ingestion of fructose was characterized by the sympathetic activation of heart accompanied by the elevation of the cardiac output and without the alteration of the total peripheral resistance. For the investigation into the same quantities of glucose, the authors stated that the ingestion of the soft drink elevated the cardiac output without a peripheral vasodilatation accompanied and the blood pressure was thus not varied. The authors subsequently concluded that diets including repeated fructose loads were likely to have a potential of resulting in increases in the risk of CVDs though it may not be easy to illustrate acute responses to long-term impacts.

There was one reported study that investigated 88,520 females at the age of 34–59 years old and the subjects did not have diabetes, strokes, or coronary heart diseases previously diagnosed in 1980 [33]. In this study, the investigating period of follow-up was from 1980 to 2004. The authors concluded that the consumption of sugar-sweetened soft drinks was positively linked to the elevation of CVD risks, whereas that of artificial sweetener-sweetened soft drinks was not. This study again showed that sugars in the soft drinks were responsible for increasing CVD risks. They did not tell what kind of artificial sweeteners were employed in making the diet soft drinks so that an appropriate comparison between the varieties of different sweeteners could not be undertaken. The authors believed that the elevation of uric acid and plasma glucose caused by the consumption of sugar-sweetened soft drinks might be the reason for increasing CVD risks. The increase in methylgloxal levels by the consumption of sugar-sweetened soft drinks might also be the reason for increasing CVD risks [13]. The methylgloxal (also called 2-oxopropanal or pyruvaldehyde) has two carbonyl groups (i.e. a ketone and an aldehyde) which are highly reactive, and it is the main pro-end product, which is toxic to tissues and cells, of the advanced glycation [34], and also positively linked to uremic states, diabetic complications, and hypertension [35].

References

[1] Yamada, M., Murakami, K., Sasaki, S., Takahashi, Y., Okubo, H., (2008). Soft drink intake is associated with diet quality even among young Japanese women with low soft drink intake. *J. Am. Diet. Assoc.* 108(12), 1997–2004.

[2] Nielsen, S.J., Popkin, B.M., (2004). Changes in beverage intake between 1977 and 2001. *Am. J. Prev. Med.* 27, 205–10.

[3] Wells, F.W., Busby, J.C., Dietary assessment of major trends in US Food Consumption, 1970–2005. Economic information bulletin no. 33: 18. United States Department of Agriculture Economic Research Service; 2008.

[4] Brown, C.M., Dulloo, A.G., Montani, J.P., (2008). Sugary drinks in the pathogenesis of obesity and cardiovascular diseases. *Intern. J. Obes.* 32, S28–S34.

[5] Murphy, S.P., Johnson, R.K., (2003). The scientific basis of recent US guidance on sugars intake. *Am. J. Clin. Nutr.* 78, 827S–833S.

[6] Aktas, A.Y., (2006). The effects of television food advertisement on children's food purchasing requests. *Pediatr. Int.* 48, 138–145.

[7] Johnston, L.D., Delva, J., O'Malley, P.M., (2007). Soft drink availability, contracts, and revenues in American secondary schools. *Am. J. Prev. Med.* 33 (4 Suppl), S209–S225.

[8] Bray, G.A., Nielsen, S.J., Popkin, B.M., (2004). Consumption of high-fructose corn syrup in beverages may play a role in the epidemic of obesity. *Am. J. Clin. Nutr.* 79, 537–543.

[9] Pepino, M.Y., Tiemann, C.D., Paterson, B.W., Wice, B.M., Klein, S., (2013). Sucralose Affects Glycemic and Hormonal Responses to an Oral Glucose Load. *Diabetes Care* 36(9), 2530-5.

[10] Liu, S., Wu, W., (2015). Dietary Safety of Leaf Sweeteners. In: W. Wu. (Ed.). Sweeteners: Resources, Processing and Health Effects. New York: Nova Science Publishers; 2015; pp.175-187.

[11] Whitehouse, R.C., Boullata, J., McCauley, L.A., (2008). The Potential Toxicity of Artificial sweeteners. *AAOHN J.* 56(6), 251-259.

[12] Bernstein, A.M., de Koning, L., Flint, A.J., Rexrode, K.M., Willett, W.C., (2012). Soda consumption and the risk of stroke in men and women. *Am. J. Clin. Nutr.* 95(5), 1190-9.

[13] Eshak, E.S., Iso, H., Kokubo, Y., Saito, S., Yamagishi, K., Inoue, M., Tsugane, S., (2012). Soft drink intake in relation to incident ischemic heart disease, stroke, and stroke subtypes in Japanese men and women: the Japan Public Health Centre–based study cohort I. *Am. J. Clin. Nutr.* 96(6), 1390-1397.

[14] Dhingra, R., Sullivan, L., Jacques, P.F., Wang, T.J., Fox, C.S., Meigs, J.B., D'Agostino, R.B., Gaziano, J.M., Vasan, R.S., (2007). Soft drink consumption and risk of developing cardiometabolic risk factors and the metabolic syndrome in middle-aged adults in the community. *Circulation* 116, 480–488.

[15] Tamez, M., López-Ridaura, R., Monge, A., Romieu, I., Rinaldi, S., Yunes, E., Blanco, M., Lajous, M., (2014). Abstract P068: Soda consumption and biomarkers of cardiovascular risk in Mexican women. *Circulation* 129, AP068.

[16] Schoppen, S., Pérez-Granados, A.M., Carbajal, A., Oubiña, P., Sánchez-Muniz, F.J., Gómez-Gerique, J.A., Vaquero, M.P., (2004). A sodium-rich carbonated mineral water reduces cardiovascular risk in postmenopausal women. *J. Nutr.* 134, 1058 –1063.

[17] Frary, C.D., Johnson, R.K., Wang, M.Q., (2005). Food sources and intakes of caffeine in the diets of persons in the United States. *J. Am. Diet. Assoc.* 105, 110–113.

[18] Winkelmayer, W.C., Stampfer, M.J., Willett, W.C., Curhan, G.C., (2005). Habitual caffeine intake and the risk of hypertension in women. *JAMA*. 294, 2330–2335.

[19] Dulloo, A.G., Miller, D.S., (1986). The thermogenic properties of ephedrine/methylxanthine mixtures: human studies. *Int. J. Obes.* 10, 467–481.

[20] Bowman, S.A., Vinyard, B.T., (2004). Fast food consumption of US adults: impact on energy and nutrient intakes and overweight status. *J. Am. Coll. Nutr.* 23, 163–168.

[21] Vogel, R.A., Corretti, M.C., Plotnick, G.D., (1997). Effect of a single high-fat meal on endothelial function in healthy subjects. *Am. J. Cardiol.* 79, 350–354.

[22] Jeppesen, J., Chen, Y.I., Zhou, M.Y., Schaaf, P., Coulston, A., Reaven, G.M., (1995). Postprandial triglyceride and retinyl ester responses to oral fat: effects of fructose. *Am. J. Clin. Nutr.* 61, 787–791.

[23] Heine, R.J., Dekker, J.M., (2002). Beyond postprandial hyperglycaemia: metabolic factors associated with cardiovascular disease. *Diabetologia* 45, 461–475.

[24] O'Keefe, J.H., Gheewala, N.M., O'Keefe, J.O., (2008). Dietary strategies for improving postprandial glucose, lipids, inflammation, and cardiovascular health. *J. Am. Coll. Cardiol.* 51, 249–255.

[25] Paolisso, G., Manzella, D., Ferrara, N., Gambardella, A., Abete, P., Tagliamonte, M.R., De Lucia, D., Furgi, G., Picone, C., Gentile, S., Rengo, F., Varricchio, M., (1997). Glucose ingestion affects cardiac ANS in healthy subjects with different amounts of body fat. *Am. J. Physiol.* 273(3Pt1), E471–E478.

[26] Paolisso, G., Manzella, D., Tagliamonte, M.R., Rizzo, M.R., Gambardella, A., Varricchio, M., (1999). Effects of different insulin infusion rates on heart rate variability in lean and obese subjects. *Metab.* 48, 755–762.

[27] Schwarz, J.M., Acheson, K.J., Tappy, L., Piolino, V., Muller, M.J., Felber, J.P., Jéquier, E., (1992). Thermogenesis and fructose metabolism in humans. *Am. J. Physiol.* 262(5 Pt 1), E591–E598.

[28] Vollenweider, P., Tappy, L., Randin, D., Schneiter, P., Jequier, E., Nicod, P., Scherrer, U., (1993). Differential effects of hyperinsulinemia and carbohydrate metabolism on sympathetic nerve activity and muscle blood flow in humans. *J. Clin. Invest.* 92, 147–154.

[29] Baron, A.D., Brechtel, G., (1993). Insulin differentially regulates systemic and skeletal muscle vascular resistance. *Am. J. Physiol.* 265 (1 Pt 1), E61–E67.

[30] Tappy, L., Randin, J.P., Felber, J.P., Chiolero, R., Simonson, D.C., Jequier, E., DeFronzo, R.A., (1986). Comparison of thermogenic effect of fructose and glucose in normal humans. *Am. J. Physiol.* 250(6 Pt 1), E718–E724.

[31] Brundin, T., Wahren, J., (1993). Whole body and splanchnic oxygen consumption and blood flow after oral ingestion of fructose or glucose. *Am. J. Physiol.* 264(4 Pt 1), E504–E513.

[32] Brown, C.M., Dulloo, A.G., Yepuri, G., Montani, J.P., (2008). Fructose ingestion acutely elevates blood pressure in healthy young humans. *Am. J. Physiol. Regul. Integr. Comp. Physiol.* 294, R730–R737.

[33] Fung, T.T., Malik, V., Rexrode, K.M., Manson, J.E., Willett, W.C., Hu, F.B., (2009). Sweetened beverage consumption and risk of coronary heart disease in women. *Am. J. Clin. Nutr.* 89, 1037–42.

[34] Ramasamy, R., Yan, S.F., Schmidt, A.M., (2006). Methylglyoxal comes of AGE. *Cell* 124, 258–60.

[35] Wang, X., Jia, X., Chang, T., Wu, L., (2008). Attenuation of hypertension development by scavenging methylglyoxal in fructose-treated rats. *J. Hypertens.* 26, 765–72.

Chapter 7

Adverse Effects of Alkaloids

Alkaloids may be biologically defined as a group of heterocyclic and active biomolecules that contain nitrogen. Most of alkaloids are naturally occurring. The structural diversity of alkaloids is great and therefore the classification of them is not commonly uniform, as compared to most other varieties of naturally occurring molecules. The naturally occurring alkaloids mainly include pyrrolidine derivatives (originating from arginine or ornithine), tropane derivatives (originating from arginine or ornithine), pyrrolizidine derivatives (originating from arginine or ornithine, L-homoserine + L-proline), piperidine derivatives (originating from lysine or octanoic acid), quinolizidine derivatives (originating from lysine), indolizidine derivatives (originating from lysine), pyridine derivatives (originating from isoleucine or nicotinic acid), isoquinoline derivatives and related alkaloids (originating from phenylalanine or tyrosine), oxazole derivatives (originating from tyrosine), isoxazole derivatives (originating from ibotenic acid), thiazole derivatives (originating from tyrosine, cysteine or 1-deoxy-D-xylulose 5-phosphate), quinazoline derivatives (originating from ornithine or phenylalanine or anthranilic acid), acridine derivatives (originating from anthranilic acid), quinoline derivatives (originating from tryptophan or anthranilic acid), indole derivatives (originating from tryptophan), imidazole derivatives (originating from histidine), purine derivatives (originating from xanthosine that is produced in purine biosynthesis), β-phenylethylamine derivatives (originating from phenylalanine or tyrosine), colchicine alkaloids (originating from phenylalanine or tyrosine), muscarine (originating from glutamic acid), benzylamine (originating from phenylalanine with isoleucine, leucine, or valine), putrescine derivatives or spermidine derivatives or spermine derivatives (originating from ornithine), peptide alkaloids with a 13- or 14- or 15-membered cycle (originating from different amino acids), diterpenes (originating from mevalonic acid), and steroids (originating from arginine, cholesterol).

The alkaloids mentioned in the above paragraph are biologically active at the various cellular levels of organisms. Some of them are important molecules that are involved in defence, agressivity, enjoy servations, or feeding, and so on. Some of the alkaloids mentioned above are quite toxic while some of them are pharmacologically active. The essential nutrients, including thiamine, riboflavin or nicotiamide may also be regarded as alkaloids. Therefore, alkaloids are very important compounds that are worth being understood.

Alkaloids are widely present in the animal or plant kingdom. They could be exogenous or endogenous in an animal body, which are different from those originating from plants. They could be found in consumer or producer chains in nature. Many alkaloids exist in commonly consumed foods. Some of them can increase CVD risks, even though they may be employed as medicines [1,2]. The aim of this chapter is to discuss those dietary alkaloids that may be associated with CVD risks.

Synephrines

The structural diagram of synephrine is shown in Figure 11. Synephrine has biological activities that are quite vital for human health. The biological activities include: resulting in the constriction of peripheral blood vessels, the dilation of pupils and the elevation of blood pressure. These biological activities may be due to that it is a stimulator (an agonist) of adrenergic receptors. The stimulating action distinctly has a preference of the α_1 to the α_2 subtype of adrenergic receptors. Nevertheless, a relatively high level of synephrine is needed to activate the α-adrenergic receptors. For example, doses of 20–100 mg by a parenteral injection are usually employed as a vasoconstrictor that is able to treat hypotension though doses of 3-30 mg by a single oral administration are generally used via dietary supplementations [7]. Its potency of stimulating β-adrenergic receptors (including all subtypes) is much weaker, as compared to that of activating α-adrenergic receptors. Synephrine also has a weak potency of interacting with trace adrenergic amine receptors and stimulating 5-HT receptors. Generally, most synephrines in the form of the l-, or R-(-)- enantiomer have stronger potencies, as compared to those in the form of the d-, or S-(+)- enantiomer though they all have been investigated. Most investigations employed a racemic mixture of the two enantiomers as a studying material.

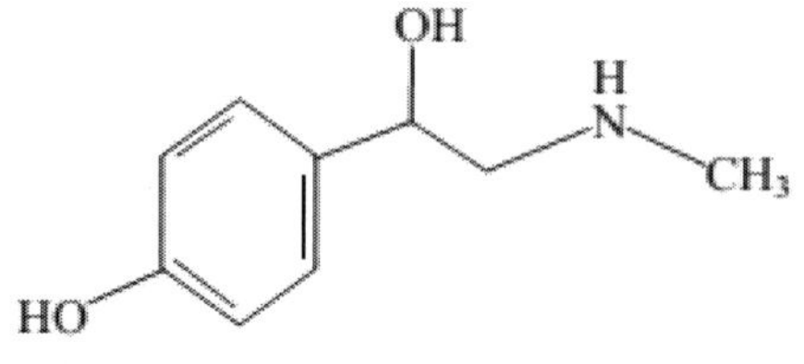

Figure 11. Structural diagram of synephrine.

Synephrine can be produced inside the human body. Its synthesis pathway in the human body is as the following: Phenylanine (also possibly starting up the pathway with this compound) → Tyrosine → tyramine → octopamine → synephrine. Therefore, synephrines at low concentrations have been detected in mammalian tissues [3,4] and in urine in a healthy human body [5,6]. The normal concentration of synephrine in human blood plasma was reported to be 0.90-13.69 ng/mL [7]. For decreasing the possibility of synephrine contributed by diets, the analysis of the urine collected from the subjects who did not consume any product of citrus for 48 h [6].

Therefore, the synephrine in the blood actually results from two sources: 1, synthesis in the body, 2, diets or foods. In a healthy body, the concentration of synephrine should be at the normal level that has been mentioned in the above paragraph. If the elevated level of synephrine detected in the blood without sufficient amounts of dietary supplements, there might be a biological dysfunction. Certain amounts of dietary synephrines ingested should increase their levels in the blood. A too high level of synephrines in the blood can cause health problems. For example, it was reported that the elevated concentration of synephrines in blood platelets (i.e. 0.72 ng/10^8 platelets) resulted in aura-associated migraine whereas the lower level of it in the blood (i.e. 0.33 ng/10^8 platelets) did not. [8].

Acute and Subchronic Toxicity of Synephrine

There were several studies that measured the acute toxicity of synephrine. The experiments on different animals or by different administration methods gave different results. When the acute toxicities of racemic synephrines measured by studying different animals are indicated as "the maximum dose tolerated " after s.c administration, the results are as the following: 400 mg/kg in guinea pig, 400 mg/kg in rat, and 300 mg/kg in mouse while they were detected to be: 500 mg/kg in guinea pigs, 500 mg/kg in rats, and 400 mg/kg in mice in case of expressed in the term of "lethal doses" [9]. The LD_{50} of synephrines was found to be 270 mg/kg by i.v. administration in mice [10].

The subchronic toxicity of synephrines has also been reported. A study found a low subchronic toxicity of synephrines in mice [11]. The authors fed the mice at doses of 30 and 300 mg/kg synephrines by an oral administration for 28 days and found that the treatment at all doses tested did not cause significant variations with hematological or biochemical parameters as well as relative organ weights except for some alterations in the level of glutathione and the activity of glutathione peroxidase.

Diets may not result in such a high level of synephrines ingested. However, the chronic effect of dietary synephrines on human health, especially the cardiovascular health, may not be ignorable.

Synephrine and CVDs

Synephrines, (also classified as ephedra alkaloids) may increase the risk of an ischemic stroke, hypertension, and a heart attack (myocardial infarction) [12] and arrhythmias [13]. A bitter orange extract containing *p*-synephrine was reported to cause significant increases in the heart rate and blood pressure [14]. Although the adverse effect of *p*-synephrine in a pure state on the cardiovascular system is not reported in the literature, other synephrines are stated to have adverse effects [15]. Furthermore, it was reported that patients with monoamine oxidase inhibitor recipients, narrow-angle glaucoma, tachyarrhythmias, and severe hypertension should not consume Seville orange juice and individuals ingesting cold preparations that contain decongestants should also avoid the consumption of Seville orange juice [16].

Controversial reports can also be found. At a dose of 25 mg/kg, a *Citrus sinensis* peel extract exhibits hypoglycemic, insulin stimulatory, antiperoxidative, antithyroidal, and cardioprotective properties and reduces the levels of cholesterols and triglycerides in the blood after daily dosing for 10 days [1,2]. Especially, a comprehensive review published in 2012 concluded that no positive association of pure *p*-synephrine (or bitter orange extract, with *p*-synephrine being the major component, alone) or combined with other herbal ingredients with the alteration of urinalysis, blood cell counts, serum chemistry or electrocardiographic data, and an elevation of blood pressure or heart rate could be reasonably predicted by the past literature [17]. Their review covered almost all the human studies including those unpublished and published in the past literature, which related to the extract of *Citrus aurantium* (bitter orange) and its primary protoalkaloid (i.e. *p*-synephrine) that were widely used and provided an assessment or information of their efficacy and safety. The authors summarized and critiqued the results of more than twenty investigations associating with about 360 individuals who ingested *p*-synephrine alone or combined with other components. The reviewed investigations included more than 50% of overweight/obese participants, and about 2/3 of the overweight/obese participants ingested caffeines (132-528 mg/day) in combination with the intake of *p*-synephrines (10-53 mg/day). The products that contained bitter orange/*p*-synephrine were administrated for up to 84 days. The proportion of the participants ingested a bitter orange/*p*-synephrine only product was about 44%, while the rest ingested a testing material that was made of the mixture of *p*-synephrines and other multiple components. The authors also concluded that *p*-synephrines alone or in conjunction with other ingredients elevated energy expenditure and resting metabolic rate, and resulted in the modest elevation of weight loss with products that contained bitter orange extract/*p*-synephrine when administrated for 42 to 84 days, and that the further assessment of their efficacy and the confirmation of their safety need longer term investigations. However, these reports did not deny the association of *p*-synephrines or bitter orange extract with ischemic strokes, myocardial infarction and arrhythmias which were indicated by other authors (see the above first paragraph of this section). Another study published in 2013, which fed Sprague–Dawley rats at a daily dosage of 10 or 50 mg of synephrine/kg body weight from one of two different bitter orange extracts by gavage for 28 days, included some doses with added caffeines and let rats run on a treadmill for 30 min/day, 3 days/week, concluded that the significant elevation of diastolic and systolic blood pressure for up to 8 hours after administration resulted from both doses of both extracts [18]. Although the authors stated that the variation of body temperature and heart rate was likely to be primarily caused by caffeines, they did not deny the association of synephrine/bitter orange extracts with an elevated diastolic and systolic blood pressure.

Therefore, it seems that there are still some uncertainties related to the association of synephrines with CVD risks. It would be worth carrying out further investigations into the cardiac toxicity of naturally occurring synephrines in the pure state.

Dietary Sources of Synephrine

Synephrine was first separated from various *Citrus* leaves and its presence in various *Citrus* juices was also recorded in the early 1960s [19]. This naturally occurring compound can now be artificially synthesized. The presence of synephrines in higher plants was investigated and the investigating results were published in 1970 [20]. It was reported that all plants of the family Rutaceae, *Zanthoxylum* [21] and *Evodia* species [22] contain synephrines. Dried *Pogostemon cablin* (Lamiaceae, patchouli) leaves contain trace amounts (0.003%) of synephrines [23]. Certain cactus species of the genera *Coryphantha* and *Dolichothele* also contain synephrines [24]. Nevertheless, sweet or bitter oranges or some other varieties of *Citrus* species are currently believed to be the predominant sources of synephrines. Some varieties of oranges may usually be included in the human diets.

The synthesis pathway of synephrines in citrus is as the following: tyrosine → tyramine → N-methyltyramine → synephrine. Tyrosine decarboxylase, tyramine N-methyltransferase and N-methyl-tyramine-β-hydroxylase are involved in the first, the second, and the third step, respectively [25,26].

The content of synephrines and its products may greatly vary with the variations of its growing area. It was found that the levels of synephrines in the products obtained by extracting from the unripe fruit of "bitter" oranges (Asian cultivars of *Citrus (C.) aurantium*), grown in China, were ca. 1 – 3 mg/g, or 0.1 - 0.3% [27]. The level of synephrines in the dried fruit of *C. aurantium* collected in Italy was found to be ca. 1 mg/g and that in its peel was found to be > 3 times higher than that in its pulp [28]. The concentrations of synephrines in sweet oranges (including Tarocco, Naveline and Navel varieties), collected from the Italian market, were reported to be ca. 13-34 μg/g (i.e. 13–34 mg/kg) while its levels in separated pulps and juices were found to be roughly the same; by calculation, these levels would supply ca. 6 mg of synephrines by ingesting one "average" Tarocco orange [29]. The concentrations of synephrines in 32 different orange "jams", the majority of them originating from the UK and US and some samples from Lebanon, Spain, Italy, or France, were found to be 0.05 mg/g - 0.0009 mg/g in bitter orange jams, and 0.05 mg/g - 0.006 mg/g in sweet orange jams [30]. The level of synephrines in *Citrus (C.) unshiu* (Satsuma mandarin) marmalade, collected in Japan, was found to be ca. 2.4 mg/20 g serving (or ca. 0.12 mg/g) [31]. The concentration of synephrines in *C. unshiu* juices that were commercial samples sold in Japan was measured to be ca. 360 mg/L (or roughly 0.36 mg/g) [31], and that in the juice made from a variety of *Satsuma* mandarin planted in California, was found to be 55 – 160 mg/L [32]. Their levels in "sweet" orange juices, bought from Brazilian markets were detected to be ca. 10 –22 mg/L while soft drinks made of oranges, commercially sold on the Brazilian market, contained an average of ca. 1 mg/L synephrines [33]. The content of synephrines in orange juices commercially sold on Italian market was found to be ca. 13–32 mg/L [34]. An investigation into more than over 50 citrus fruit juices (both hand-squeezed and commercially-prepared juices of fresh fruits), bought from the US market, indicated ca 4 – 60 mg/L of synephrine content while it was not detectable in the juices of lemon, lime or grapefruits [30]. The content of synephrines in the juices that were produced by using fresh, peeled fruits of various citrus, was found to be as the following: Ugli tangelo (*C. reticulate* × *C. paradisi*), ca. 47 mg/kg; Meyer lemon (*C. limon* Tan.), ca. 3 mg/kg; clementine (*C. clementina* Tan.), ca. 115 mg/L; Nova tangerine (*C. reticulate* Tan.), ca. 78 mg/L; Marrs sweet orange (*C. sinensis* Tan.), ca. 85 mg/L whereas that in Wekiwa tangelo (*C. reticulate* × *C. paradisi*), Red-fleshed pummelo (*C. grandis* Tan.), and Rio Red grapefruit (*C. paradise* Macf.) was found to be not detectable [35]. Synephrines with structural similarities includes *p*-synephrine, *m*-synephrine, ephedrine, norepinephrine, epinephrine, and amphetamine. Until now, synephrines are mainly found to be present in citrus fruits and juices (especially in *C. aurantium*), 90% of synephrines being *p*-synephrine [15].

Caffeine

Caffeine is biologically active. The biological activity of caffeine should originate from its chemical properties. Caffeine may be classified as a xanthine alkaloid. An imidazole and a pyrimidinedione comprise two fused rings (the xanthine core) (see Figure 12). The two functional groups of pyrimidinedione are amides, which are predominately present in a zwitterionic resonance (the position from which the amide carbon atoms are connected to their adjacent nitrogen atoms by double bonds). Therefore, in the ring system of pyrimidinedione, the six atoms comprising the ring are planar and sp^2 hybridized. According to Hückel's rule, the fused 5,6 ring core of caffeine is aromatic because it totally has ten π electrons [36].

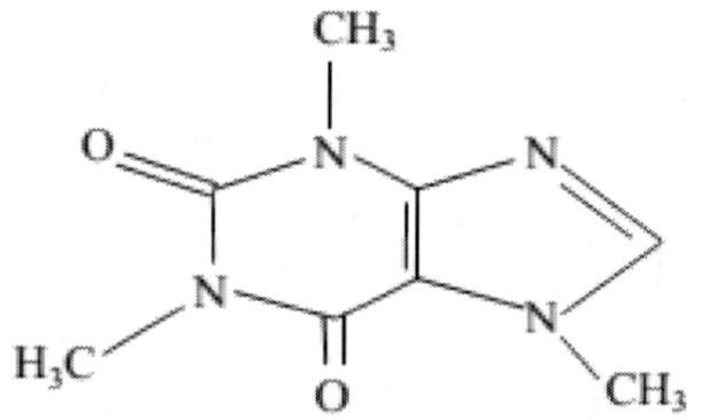

Figure 12. Structural diagram of caffeine.

Purified caffeine is odorless and its taste is slightly bitter. It could be a white soft powder or crystal and its melting point is ca. 235–238°C. The solubility of caffeine in water is moderate (ca. 2 g/100 mL at room temperature) and very high in boiling water (66 g/100 mL) while its solubility in ethanol is also moderate (1.5 g/100 mL) [37]. Caffeine is a weakly basic compound (pK_a = ca. 0.6) and its protonation needs a strong acid [38]. There is not any stereogenic centers in a caffeine molecule [39] and caffeine is considered as an achiral molecule [40].

There are >25 metabolites (mainly Theophylline, Theobromine and Paraxanthine) that result from the metabolism of caffeine in humans [41]. Paraxanthine accounts for 72 to 80% of the final metabolites resulted from the metabolism of caffeine. Caffeine metabolism in adults is associated with five major metabolic pathways [42, 43]. The first three are composed of N-7, N-1, and N-3 demethylizations to produce Theophylline (a muscular, bronchiole, vascular, and respiratory relaxant), Theobromine (causing the elevation of muscular and cerebral blood flow, a vasodilator) and Paraxanthine, respectively. The three demethylizations involve the hepatic cytochrome P-450 isoenzyme that metabolizes 95% caffeines, which result in an average *in vivo* metabolism rate of 5% theophyllines, 10% theobromines, and 85% paraxanthines [44]. The production of uracil metabolites results from the fourth pathway while the fifth pathway is that the rest part of caffeines, whicht is un-degraded in the process, is eliminated in the renal. Variations in metabolism are the main reasons for the large inter-individual variation of the plasmatic level of caffeines after administrating the same dose. There are four factors caused the differences: the occurrence of liver diseases, individuality (sex, weight), metabolic inhibition and the induction of cytochrome P-450, and the polymorphisms of genes [43]. The absorption of caffeines from the intestinal tract is quickly and completely, so that its bioavailability is 100%. The time for reaching the maximum level in plasma (Tmax) was reported to be 30 – 45 minutes [45, 43, 46, 47] after administration and the consumption of foods can delay it while its average metabolic half life in humans was reported to be 2.5 - 4.5 hours [48].

Caffeine can be produced by employing malonic acid and dimethylurea as starting materials [49,50]. No report indicates that it can be synthesized in the human body. However, it is rarely produced by artificial manufacturing. And also, an artificially produced caffeine is rarely employed in making food products or included in human diets. Human beings mainly consume natural caffeines which originate from food or beverage products made from natural materials that contain it and sometimes that added to the food or beverage products.

Dietary Sources of Caffeine

There are many plant species or varieties (ca. 60) with the presence of caffeines. However, coffee beans or seeds, kola nuts and tea leaves may be the most common sources of caffeines. The leaves of Amazonian holly guayusa, South American holly yerba mate and yaupon holly, and the seeds of Amazonian maple guarana berries are the other sources of caffeines. In temperate area worldwide, there are also unrelated caffeine-containing varieties of plants. Some beverages or foods and its products may have different effects on human health even with the same content of caffeines. This may be caused by the fact that caffeine-containing plants may also be rich in polyphenols that can interact with caffeines to produce precipitates and other methylxanthine alkaloids (such as theobromine and theophylline that have a cardiac stimulating activity).

Coffees, caffeine tablets, energy drinks, chocolates, soft drinks (e.g. colas), teas, other beverages, inhalations and the oral products may contain caffeines [51]. The main sources of caffeines include coffee beans (0.8-2.5%), tea leaves (ca. 4%), guarana seeds (2-4.5%), and Cola nuts (2-3.5%) [52]. Another report stated that the caffeine content of coffee beans may be 1.3 to 2.4% (dry weight) [53].

The dietary consumption of caffeines primarily results from coffee drinking, one of the most popular beverages that are frequently consumed worldwide. Generally, the content of caffeines in coffee may vary greatly with the variation of the preparation technique, the type of coffee beans, growing conditions, even the parts of harvesting beans in a coffee tree, etc. Depending upon the beans/water ratio employed in making a coffee drink, the amount of ingested caffeine from one serving may vary a lot.

Drinking tea is another dietary source of caffeines. Tea is also one of the most frequently consumed beverages in the world. The content (by dry weight) of caffeines in tea is higher than that in coffee. However, a typical serving of tea may supply less caffeines, as compared to that of coffee because coffee is normally prepared stronger than tea. The variation of processing procedures or methods, growing conditions, and other factors may also result in the variation of content of caffeines in tea. Therefore, there may be more caffeines in certain types of tea than in other types of tea [54]. For example, the authors also stated that the caffeine content of teas like the pale Japanese green tea, *gyokuro* is far higher than that of much darker teas like *lapsang souchong* that only has very small amounts of caffeines.

Caffeine is also employed as a common additive in making soft drinks, for example cola that was initially made from kola nuts. The amount of caffeines added to the soft drinks may vary with different manufacturers and 12 ounce serving of it may typically supply 9 - 70 mg caffeines. The level of caffeines in the soft drinks outside the range mentioned above might not be ruled out. By comparison, some energy drinks might supply more than 81 mg caffeines per serving. The energy drink employed Guarana as a prime component could supply large quantities of caffeines accompanied with small quantities of theophyllines and theobromines in a naturally occurring slow-release excipient [55].

Only small quantities of caffeines are present in chocolates made from cocoa beans. Chocolate has a weak stimulant effect that may result from a combination of caffeines, theophyllines, and theobromines [56].

There are other artificially made tablets or products or inhalations sold in the market. However, this kind of caffeine sources may not be dietetically important. So they are not introduced in detail here.

Acute Toxicity of Caffeine

The over-intake or overdose of caffeines can cause caffeine intoxication (i.e. the over-stimulation of central nervous system) [57]. The symptoms caused by the overdose of caffeines are quite similar to that caused by the over-intake of other stimulants: possibly including psychomotor agitation, irregular or rapid heart beat, irritability, a rambling flow of thought and speech, muscle twitching, gastrointestinal disturbance, an increased urination, the flushing of the face, insomnia, excitement, anxiety, fidgeting, and restlessness [58]. The toxicity is however caused by the dose that is much higher than the amount of caffeines supplied by common caffeinated drinks or tablets (such as an ingestion of > 250 mg at a time) [59]. When much higher overdoses of caffeines occur, psychosis, hallucinations, delusions, disinhibition, disorientation, lapses in judgment, depression, and mania may be observed and the development of rhabdomyolysis (broken skeletal muscle tissue) can occur [60].

Death can be caused by an extreme overdose of caffeines. The LD_{50} of caffeines in humans varies with the variation of sensitivity of individuals. It was reported to be ca. 150 - 200 mg/kg body weight or ca. 70 - 100 cups of coffee for an average adult [61-64].

For these high doses of caffeine, a damaged liver is usually observed. It seems no report on a damaged cardiovascular system that is caused by the acute toxicity of caffeine overdose can be found in the past literature except for irregular or rapid heart beat.

This high dose of caffeines is very unlikely to be caused by an ordinary diet. Both foods and beverages are unlikely to supply a sufficient amount of caffeines which can result in the acute toxicity.

Caffeine and CVDs

There are many reports involving epidemiological studies that stated the positive association of regular ingestion of caffeines with CVDs in the past literature. However, this suggestion is not proven by some other's studies and some comprehensive reviews recently published. What is the truth?

Caffeine appears to be consistently reported on its capacity of significantly elevating blood pressure and other CVD outcomes [65-73]. Its ability to antagonize adenosine receptors and oppose the actions of adenosine may be involved in the mechanism of caffeine toxicity that may vary with different genotypes. It was suggested that the effect of caffeines on blood pressure via the inhibition of adenosine receptors and an elevated release of select neurotransmitters [74]. A paper published in 2012 concluded that the acute administration of caffeines resulted in the variation of wave reflections in healthy participants, the promotion of arterial stiffness, and the elevation of blood pressure [75]. This result is consistent with those reported in the past literature which stated that the ingestion of caffeines resulted in hypertension (especially the elevation of aortic pressure) and elevated the aortic stiffness in healthy adults [75-80]. Furthermore, caffeine may adversely affect the cardiovascular system ranging from a moderate increase in heart rate to more severe cardiac arrhythmias [81] and acutely increase arterial stiffness [82]. Caffeine plus ephedrine could increase the risk of myocardial necrosis and an irregular heart rate [83]. Caffeine (1-5 mg/kg) increased the incidence of both supraventricular and ventricular arrhythmias [84].

Controversially, the consumption of caffeinated drinks has been reported to be not associated with arrhythmias or have a lower risk of incident arterial stiffness [85,86]. This may be explained by the toxicity of caffeines which may be dependent upon its concentration since its concentration at less than 0.58% extended life span, but higher than 0.58% shortened life span [87]. Nevertheless, these reports did not deny the positive association of consumption of caffeines with the elevation of blood pressure, myocardial necrosis and an irregular heart rate, which were stated by other authors mentioned in the above paragraph of this section. One report just reviewed the studies on patients with known arrhythmias [86]. There were also several reports that stated the development of tolerance to its physiological impacts on hormonal reactivity and blood pressure led by the habitual use of caffeines [88-90]. A review paper published in 2014 stated that the consumption of coffee is not positively associated with CVD mortalities, heart failures, strokes, and coronary heart diseases [91]. This review did not cover the association of caffeines with other CVDs. Furthermore, other components in the coffee may be beneficial for the cardiovascular system.

Tyramine

It has been reported that tyramine exists in several areas of the human brain [92]. Its structural diagram is shown in Figure 13. Tyramine can be biochemically synthesized via the decarboxylation of tyrosine, which is enzymatically catalyzed by tyrosine decarboxylase [93,94].

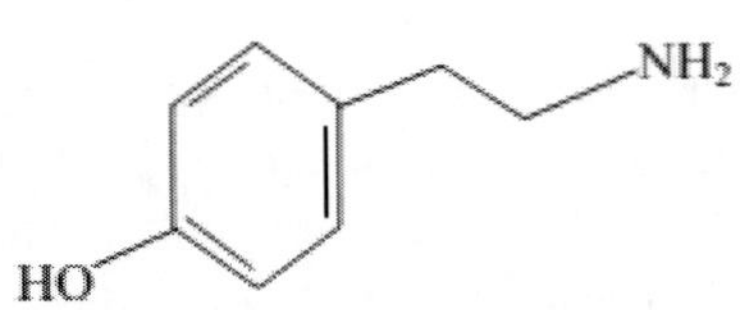

Figure 13. Structural diagram of tyramine.

The discovery of high affinity of a trace amine-associated receptor (a G protein-coupled receptor) for a tyramine indicated its possibility of biologically acting as a neurotransmitter [95,96]. The presence of the trace amine-associated receptor in peripheral tissues (including the kidneys) and the brain has been found [97]. The biological or biochemical function of tyramines is found to be associated with the release of catecholamine. It is believed that the dietary tyramine only has nonpsychoactive peripheral sympathomimetic effects, because it can not cross the blood-brain barrier. It seems that no report on whether the neurological action of tyramines has any effect on the cardiovascular system or not could be found in the past literature. There are some reports that stated the positive association of dietary tyramines with CVD risks in the literature.

Tyramine and CVDs

The over-consumption of tyramine-rich foods in combination with monoamine oxidase inhibitors would be able to cause a hypertensive crisis. Physiologically, the metabolism of tyramine needs monoamine oxidase A. If there are monoamine oxidase inhibitors in humans, the monoamine oxidase A can not be activated so that the metabolism of tyramine ingested can be impaired. Furthermore, the tyramine inside the human body is able to transfer the stored monoamines, for example, epinephrines, norepinephrines and dopamines from pre-synaptic vesicles. At this point, certain amounts of ingesting foods high in tyramines would be able to cause a hypertensive crisis. This symptom was first observed by a neurologist whose wife had severely suffered from headaches when she ate cheeses and at the same time was treated by using monoamine oxidase inhibitors [98]. Deriving from this observation, "cheese crisis" or "cheese effect" is still used for expressing the hypertensive crisis though this health problem can also be caused by ingesting other foods rich in tyramines [99]. The content of tyramines in most processed cheeses is not high enough to result in hypertensive effects, but that in aged cheeses (such as Stilton) is possibly high enough [100].

Tyramines were also reported to cause acute anterior myocardial infarction with atrial fibrillation [101]. Cardiac arrhythmias occurred in drug-free physically healthy patients with depression at a dosage as little as 0.03 mg/kg of tyramines before and after 30 mmHg elevations in systolic blood pressure [102]. A mild adverse event was caused by 6 mg tyramines in one or two usual servings, while a severe adverse event in those taking monoamine oxidase inhibitor drugs resulted from doses of 10–25 mg [103,104]. Doses of 200–800 mg dietary tyramines induced a 30 mm Hg rise in blood pressure [103].

In addition, a paper published in 2012 concluded that tyramines induced spontaneous atrial fibrillation in canine atria with elevated sympathetic nerve sprouting [105]. In this study, the authors treated experimental dogs with the perfusion of tyramines (5 μM). After treating for 42 – 56 days, 5 of 6 atria developed atrial fibrillation by tyramines whereas the control did not. An early after-depolarization-mediated triggered activity initiated the atrial fibrillation during the late phase 3. The late phase 3 early after-depolarization-mediated triggered activity arose from the junction of the left atrial pulmonary veins, which resulted in atrial fibrillation, reentry and the block of functional conduction in left atria. The mixed reentrant and focal mechanisms subsequently maintained the atrial fibrillation. The Ca_i^{2+} level being 64 ± 12% of the peak systolic Ca_i^{2+} transient amplitude resulted from simultaneous lengthening of the Ca_i^{2+} transient duration and the shortening of the action potential duration that were caused by tyramines might result in the late phase 3 early after-depolarization-mediated triggered activity. The significant elevation of growth associated protein 43 positive nerve sprouts and tyrosine hydroxylase were significantly increased in the sinus node in the tyramine treated group. If these findings by the authors [105] are true, they might be applicable for the association of tyramines with CVDs in humans.

Dietary Sources and Recommendation of Tyramine

The tyramine is widely present in animal and plant food resources [105]. Its presence in foods mainly results from the decarboxylation of tyrosine because of decay (e.g. too long storage) or fermentation. Considerable quantities of tyramines could be present in the following foods: fermented foods (e.g. an array of cacti, yeasts, processed meats, coconuts, Brazil nuts, peanuts, raspberries, red plums, figs, pineapples, bananas, avocados, edamames, snow peas, Italian flat (Romano) beans, green bean pods, broad (fava) beans, kimchi, sauerkraut, miso soups, tempeh, teriyaki sauces, soybean condiments, soy sauces, shrimp paste, yogurt, sour cream, and most cheeses, alcoholic beverages, chocolates, most porks, and meats which are marinated, fermented, smoked, aged, pickled, or spoiled [106].

The Austrian maximum tolerable levels for tyramines for foods (high consumption scenario: female user, 60 kg body mass, 95 percentile) are 1000 mg/kg for cheeses; 2000 mg/kg for fermented/raw cured meats; 950 mg/kg for fishes (raw or processed), and 800 mg/kg for sauerkrauts, which were estimated according to the local habitual consumption of these foods [107].

Dopamine

Dopamine is named according to its chemical structure (see Figure 14). The removal of a carboxyl group in a L-DOPA molecule can produce dopamine. It is a neurotransmitter of families of phenethylamine and catecholamine, and a hormone (a Prolactin Inhibiting Hormone/Factor). Therefore, it is involved in various biological or biochemical actions in the human brain and other tissues of the body.

Dopamine can be synthesized mainly in cells located in neurons and the medulla of the adrenal glands in humans. Its synthesis pathway may be as the following: L-Phenylalanine → L-Tyrosine → L-DOPA → Dopamine. The production and functions of dopamines in peripheral areas are largely independent of those in the brain since it can not cross the blood–brain barrier.

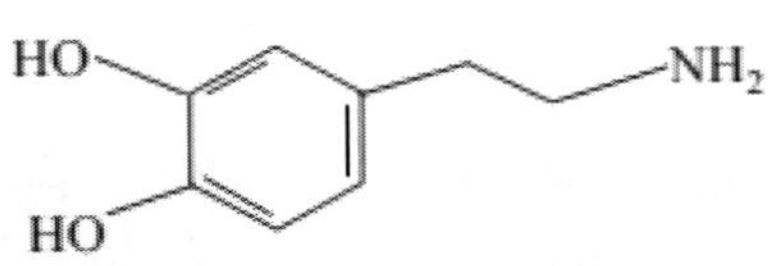

Figure 14. Structural diagram of dopamine.

Dopamine and CVDs

Dopamine is usually employed in treating cardiac arrest, circulatory shock, bradycardia (a slow heart rate) and severe hypotension, particularly in newborn infants. This application arises from its ability, which is dosage dependent, of elevating blood pressure, heart rate, urine output, and sodium excretion by the kidneys. The elevation of blood pressure and output can be achieved by the elevation of heart rate and heart muscle contraction force via 5 to 10 μg/kg/min of dopamine injection and the further elevation of blood pressure can be achieved by the elevation of vasoconstriction via 10 to 20 μg/kg/min of dopamine injection which however has adverse side effects for example causing cardiac arrhythmias and a dysfunction of kidneys [109,110]. The dose of 2 - 5 μg/kg/min of dopamine injection was reported to be not effective and sometimes might be harmful [111]. Dopamine hydrochloride-containing preparations are employed in treating septic shock, myocardial infarction, kidney failure, acute heart failure, and so on, which are on the World Health Organization's List of Essential Medicines [112].

The deficiency of dopamines in the mesolimbic system is associated with obesity [113]. Intrarenal dopamine deficiency can lead to hypertension and a decreased longevity in mice [114].

Excessive dopamines present in the body caused by injection may induce anginal pain, ventricular arrhythmias, which could be life-threatening, and an increase in heart rate [115]. The authors found that the intravenous injection of dopamines ≥ 20-40 μg/kg/min caused severe arrhythmias in the electrocardiagram occurred.

It appears to be that no report on CVDs resulting from an over-intake of dopamines could be found in the literature. However, those studies mentioned in the above paragraphs of this section may predict that both the over-loading and deficiency of dopamines in the blood would be harmful to the cardiovascular system.

Dietary Sources and Abnormality of Dopamine

Extensive literature search seems that there is no report on the association of dietary dopamines with CVD risks. However, dietary dopamines should affect their levels in the blood since they are easy to be absorbed. The association of dietary dopamines with CVDs shouldn't be ignored since the level of blood dopamines is found to be associated with CVDs.

Normally, the dopamine is degraded by oxidation which is catalyzed by monoamine oxidase in the mitochondria of many tissues. However, there are two cases that might cause health problems.

First, the intake of some drugs (e.g. the inhibitors of monoamine oxidase for treating depression) can block the degradation of dopamines. This would cause an overloading of dopamines in the blood. In this case, patients should be advised to limit or even avoid the foods that can greatly increase blood dopamines. Second, the dopamine is able to be autoxidized (i.e. directly reacting with oxygen), which forms various free radicals and quinones [116]. These chemical compounds are toxic to cells and therefore cause health problems. These two cases mentioned above indicate that the consumption of foods capable of causing the over-loading of dopamines in the blood or their over-intake should be avoided.

The intake of dopamines may affect their levels in the blood, but perhaps not in the brain since they do not cross the blood–brain barrier. The intake of L-DOPA should be able to affect the level of dopamines in both the brain and other tissues since it is a precursor for dopamine and crosses the blood–brain barrier. The intake of tyrosines (the precursor of L-DOPA) and phenylalanines (the precursor for tyrosine) could also affect the level of dopamines in both the brain and other tissues.

The dopamine is present in fava or broad beans, snow peas, bananas, and more. The maximum concentrations of dopamines found in *Vicia faba* were 10,000-20,000 mg/kg (dry weight; 100 mg/kg by wet weight) [117] while their levels can vary from 25 to100 mg/kg in bananas pulp and 800-5600 mg/kg in bananas skin [118]. The level of dopamines in Brussels sprouts, broccoli, avocados, and potatoes is ≥ 1 part per million while that in beans, spinaches, tomatoes, oranges, and other plants is < 1 part per million [119]. Dopamines in the marine green alga *Ulvaria obscura* (a major component of some algal blooms) were estimated to be as high as 4.4% of dry mass (120).

The bean pods and leaves of the genus *Mucuna* plants (particularly *Mucuna pruriens* (velvet beans)) have high content of L-DOPA [120]. The L-DOPA is also quite rich in *Vicia faba* beans (or called broad beans). However, its concentration is much higher in the pod shells and other parts of the plant than in the beans [122]. There are substantial quantities of L-DOPA in the seeds of *Bauhinia*and *Cassia* trees [123].

Serotonin

The serotonin is also named 5-hydroxytryptamine (5-HT), which is a neurotransmitter. Its structural diagram is shown in Figure 15. It is mainly situated in the gastrointestinal tract and central nervous system in humans. The serotonin found in the enterochromaffin cells in the gut (for regulating the movements of intestine) accounts for ca. 90% of its total content in the human body while the rest is secreted from the serotonergic neurons of the central nervous system (for regulating sleep, appetite and mood (a contributor to the feelings of happiness and well-being)[124]) [125]. The serotonin secreted moves out of tissues and blood platelets take up it and store it. In case of binding to a clot, platelets disgorge serotonins. The disgorged serotonin acts as a vasoconstrictor and an assistant of regulating blood clotting and hemostasis. The serotonin can also act as a growth factor of some cells and therefore may be associated with wound healing. These may be the basis of their association with cardiovascular health.

The serotonin originates from L-tryptophan (an essential amino acid). The production of serotonins in humans involves a pathway that is metabolically short and needs two enzymes (i.e. amino acid decarboxylase and tryptophan hydroxylase). The pathway is limited by the reaction catalyzed by tryptophan hydroxylase. There are two forms of tryptophan hydroxylase (1 and 2). Tryptophan hydroxylase 1 exists in various tissues whereas tryptophan hydroxylase 2 is an isoform specifically existing in the brain [126].

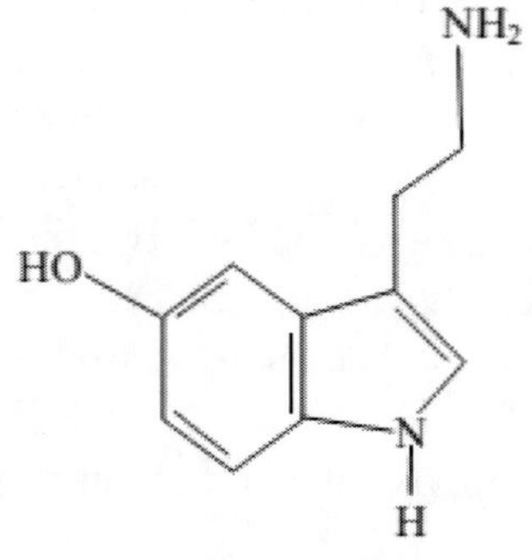

Figure 15. Structural diagram of serotonine.

Serotonin and CVDs

The deficiency of serotonins may cause depression or stress that is associated with obesity and CVDs. Furthermore, it was reported that the development of progressively losing heart strength early on was observed in mice with the deficiency of tryptophan hydroxylase 1 caused by a genetical alteration and the mice had the symptom of breathing difficulties and a pale skin, easily tired, and ultimately died because of the heart failure [126].

On the other hand, doses of 100-200 mg/kg body weight caused a serotonin syndrome (intoxication) in lab animals when administered in isolation, though no reports on toxicity at doses of ≤50 mg/kg body weight could be found [127]. Furthermore, the observation of fibrosis, especially cardiac valve fibrosis and the syndrome of retroperitoneal fibrosis caused by some serotonergic agonist drugs [128] may also indicate the association of over-activity of serotonins with CVDs. The serotonin is a vasoconstrictor, the over-intake of which may be harmful to patients with hypertension.

Dietary Sources and Abnormality of Serotonin

Generally, it is believed that serotonins do not cross the blood–brain barrier. If this is true, the intake of serotonins may only affect their levels in the blood, but perhaps not in the brain. However, some reports stated that increased serotonins can cross the blood–brain barrier. For example, it was found that augmented brain serotonins were able to cross the blood–brain barrier via the transporter of serotonins from the brain to the circulating blood [129]. Does augmented serotonins derived from the intestine cross the blood–brain barrier from the circulating blood to the brain? This question might be partially answered by the fact that the lack of serotonin synthesis in the brain was found to be partially compensated by the serotonin from the intestine [130].

Normally, dietary serotonins are unlikely to cause the over-loading of serotonins in the blood or brain since the body has a mechanism of metabolizing the un-used part of them mainly in the liver into 5-hydroxyindoleacetic acid that is excreted by the kidneys. The serotonin metabolism is catalyzed by monoamine oxidases. However, the inhibition of the enzymes in combination with the intake of serotonins would be able to result in CVD risks and perhaps other health problems.

There are two dietary sources that can increase the blood level of serotonins. One is the high intake of serotonins by eating foods since they are easy to be absorbed. Another is the high intake of their precursor, L-tryptophan which is an essential nutrient. L-tryptophan and its metabolite (5-hydroxytryptophan) are able to cross the blood–brain barrier.

Serotonin concentrations were 25–400 mg/kg in walnuts and hickory nuts, 3–30 mg/kg in plantains, pineapples, banana fruits, kiwifruits, plums, and tomatoes, and 0.1–3 mg/kg in a wide range of tested vegetables [131]. The authors also reported that the dietary over-intake of serotonins is the suspected factor of causing endomyocardial fibrosis, but which is currently not confirmed. Other foods such as mushrooms and chocolates also contain serotonins.

It should also be noted that the serotonin is synthesized from a tryptophan. So, foods high in tryptophan content may result in a high level of serotonins in the human brain and blood.

Study on the effect of dietary serotonins on the human cardiovascular system seems to be inadequate, which should be worthy to be focused on in the future.

The tryptophan was found to be present in chocolates that contained varying amounts of cocoa. The highest level (13.27–13.34 μg/g) of tryptophans was found in 70–85% cocoa [132]. Peanuts, the meats of turkey, chicken and tuna fish, breads, cheeses, milk, dried prunes, bananas, and oats are also the common sources of tryptophans [133,134]. Typically, many individuals have ca. 900 to 1000 mg daily intake of tryptophans while 250 mg/day [135,136] to 425 mg/day [137,138], which is equivalent to a daily ingestion of 3.5 - 6.0 mg/kg of the body weight, were recommended. The ingestion of alcohol (0.8g/kg of body weight) was found to reduce tryptophans by 20-25%, resulting in a similar reduction of serotonins [139,140].

Histamine

The histamine is associated with the regulation of the physiological function in the gut and local immune responses, which also acts as a neurotransmitter [141]. It also participates in inflammatory responses. Its structural diagram is shown in Figure 16.

A histamine is synthesized via the decarboxylation of a histidine (an essential amino acid). L-histidine decarboxylase catalyzes this synthesis. Granules in white blood cells (including eosinophils and basophils) and in mast cells are the main sites where most histamines are synthesized. The sites (blood vessels, the surfaces of the internal body, feet, mouth, and nose) of the potential injury are particularly rich in mast cells. There are also histamines released from non-mast cells in several tissues (including the brain). In the brain, the histamine acts as a neurotransmitter.

The enterochromaffin-like cell of the stomach is another vital site that releases and stores histamines. An immunologic reaction is the most vital way of releasing histamines from a basophil and mast cell. The proper antigen induces the attachment of IgE antibodies to the membranes of basophils and mast cells which then degranulate and release histamines. Some other alkaloids (e.g., curare alkaloids and morphine that are usually employed as drugs) are able to transfer histamines in the granules of these cells, which induce their releases. The release of histamines can also be stimulated by antibiotics (e.g. polymyxin). Histamines increase the permeability of the capillaries to white blood cells and some proteins are elevated by histamines and therefore are able to refrain pathogens from expanding to the un-infected tissues [142]. The histamine is also an amine that is vasoactive and hydrophilic. These biological or biochemical actions of histamines may be the basis of their association with CVD risks and other health problems.

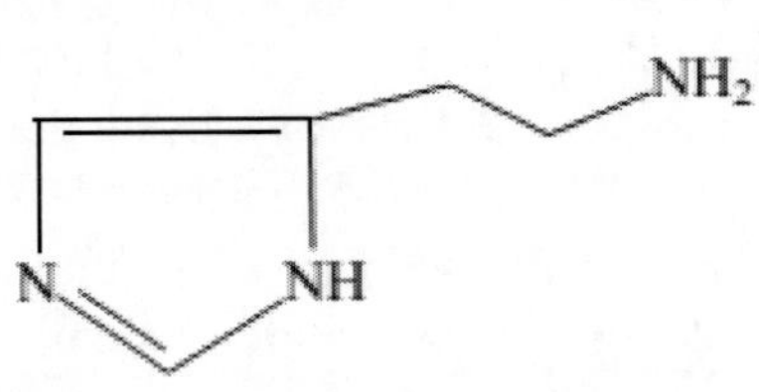

Figure 16. Structural diagram of histamine.

Histamine and CVDs

The histamine is a central nervous system (CNS) neurotransmitter and a vasodilator. Excessive histamines may cause myocardial damage, and arrhythmias, though further study is needed to illustrate their exact roles in the early stages of CVDs such as myocardial ischaemia or atherosclerosis [143]. The consumption of fishes containing histamines at <50 mg/kg, 50-200 mg/kg, 200, and 1000 mg/kg was considered to be safe, possibly toxic, probably toxic, and toxic, respectively [144]. Furthermore, it was found that the expression of adhesion molecules in vascular endothelial cells can be enhanced by histamines and therefore result in the elevation of leukocyte-endothelial cell interactions which are vital for the onset of atherogenesis [145]. The histamine was found to be a biogenic amine that reduces the expression of the hepatic LDL receptor and plasma HDLC in rats [146]. This appears to indicate the involvement of histamines in the lipoprotein metabolism that might be associated with the occurrence of atherosclerosis. It was also found that the migration and proliferation of smooth muscle cells were elevated by histamines, which were associated with atherogenesis and intimal thickening [147]. There is another report stated that the histamine was an additional index of cardiac specific enzymes and myocardial ischemia which might be a good single prognostic marker for the degree of ischemic heart diseases [148].

Other symptoms of the histamine toxicity, which is often observed, include erythemata, skin flushes, palpitations, headaches and others [149]. Among those symptoms, palpitations and headaches may be associated with the disorder of th cardiovascular system.

Dietary Sources and Abnormality of Histamine

The human body has a mechanism of quickly degrading un-used histamines. Diamine oxidases or histamine-N-methyltransferases catalyze the degradation reaction of histamines. The histamine-N-methyltransferase is the primary enzyme that catalyzes the degradation of histamines in the synapses in the central nervous system of the brain. Therefore, a normal diet or food is unlikely to result in adverse effects on human health. However, individuals who have low activity of diamine oxidases are at the risk of toxicity of histamines.

Furthermore, the absorption of histamines in the intestine is quite poor so that the ingestion of large quantities of histamine contaminated fishes may not necessarily result in any toxic effect in a health person [149]. However, if there is an intestinal lesion or disorder, the absorption of histamines becomes very easy. Very high intake of histamines could result in a great increase in its level in blood circulation.

The blood-brain barrier is not crossed by histamines [150]. Therefore, the intake of histamines should not affect their levels in the brain and subsequently cause vasoactive effects from the brain. However, L-histidines cross the blood-brain barrier. Therefore, the high intake of foods rich in histidines would greatly elevate the level of histamines in both the brain and other tissues. In this case, a health problem could be caused.

Generally, histamine levels in fresh foods may be quite low. However, its content can increase with the prolongation of storing and leaving to mature. This compound widely exists in many foods, which is shown in Table 7. Some microorganisms that may grow in aged or spoiled fishes are able to produce histamines. For example, *Photobacterium psychrotolerans, Photobacterium phosphoreum, Morganella psychrotolerans, Klebsiella pneumonia,*

Morganella morganii, and Hafnia alvei are the microorganisms that have the most ability to produce histamines, which were found in scombroid fishes that caused poisoning incidents [151-154]. *Lactobacillus curvatus, Lactobacillus buchnerii, Lactobacillus hilgardii, Lactobacillus saerimneri 30a, Lactobacillus parabuchneri or Lactobacillus rossiae, Tetragenococcus species, Leuconostoc species, Pediococcus damnosus, Pediococcus parvalus, and Oenococcus oeni* are also able to produce histamines, which were found in fermented foods or beverages [155-160].

The L-histidine is rich in some food proteins, such as beef (4.3 g/100 g protein) and eel meat proteins (4.6 g/100 g protein). It is generally considered as an essential amino acid. It seems that no report on CVDs caused by the dietary intake of histidines can be found in the past literature. However, the extra high intake of histidines in combination with the high intake of histamines and the low activity of diamine oxidases could be a risk for an adverse effect on human health.

Table 7. Histamine content in some selected foods or drinks [161]

Foods or drinks	Histamine content (mg/kg)
Red wine, champagne, white wine, beer	ca. 3.6 and 3.7
Aged (or smoked, or canned) fishes	348-8900
Fishes (tuna, mackerel, sardines, anchovy, herring, catfish, salmon), pizza, smoked and processed meats (salami, ham, bratwurst, bacon)	3.9 – 23.6
Fish sauces	96 – 197
Sauerkraut, certain vegetables (tomato, spinach, eggplant, avocado, mushrooms)	2.9 – 42.6

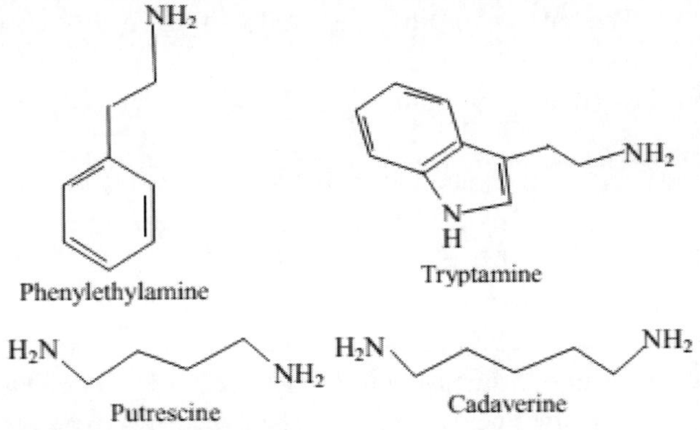

Figure 17. Structural diagram of phenylethylamine, tryptamine, putrescine and cadaverine.

Table 8. Some food or beverage products rich in putrescine [161]

Food or Beverage Categories	Putrescine Content	Food or Beverage Categories	Putrescine Content
White wine (sparkling)	5.2 mg/L	Fermented sausages	84.2 – 84.6 mg/kg
Red wine	4.2 – 4.8 mg/L	Fermented vegetables	264 mg/kg
Beer	3.3 – 3.5 mg/L	Cheeses	25.4 – 65 mg/kg
Fish sauces	98.1 – 99.3 mg/kg	Fermented fishes	13.4 – 17 mg/kg
Other savoury sauces	6 – 13.6 mg/kg		

Other Amines

There are also some other amines that are biogenic. They are derived from amino acids. They can also be synthesized in the human body, having physiological effects. They can also be produced in microorganisms. Here, putrescine, cadaverine, phenylethylamine, and tryptamine are briefly introduced. Their structural diagrams are shown in Figure 17.

Putrescine

The putrescine can be synthesized in humans, other animals or microorganisms. It can be produced by the decarboxylation of an ornithine (a free non-protein amino acid), which is catalyzed by an enzyme ornithine decarboxylase. And also, it can be synthesized from an arginine via agmatine and carbamylputrescine [162]. There is another way of producing putrescines. In this way, putrescines are produced during the biosynthesis of de novo polyamines [163].

The putrescine is the precursor of polyamines (i.e. spermine and spermidine) that are physiologically associated with the regulation of tumor promotion, cell division, and cell growth in humans [164]. It is a vital part of all mammals cells and is associated essentially with various regulating steps during the proliferation of malignant, adaptive, and normal cells. Because the proliferation rates of the colonic and intestinal mucosa are high, putrescines are especially required [165]. A new incorporation of putrescines was found to stimulate the growth of tumor in murine colon cells [166].

Dietary putrescines can be easily absorbed and a passive diffusion might be the driving force of its absorption. The putrescine in ingested foods is readily absorbed from the gut lumen in rats. It was found that the conversion rate of the absorbed putrescines into nonpolyamine metabolites (mainly into amino acids) and other polyamines was more than 80% [163].

Un-used (or extra) putrescines are degraded to aldehydes via oxidization, which is catalyzed by diamine oxidases [167]. The low activity of diamine oxidases in humans in combination with the high intake of putrescines would be likely to result in adverse effects.

The ability of putrescines to cause health problems (including illness in the cardiovascular system) appears to be not as strong as that of tyramines and histamines. It is probable that the adverse effect of dietary putrescines is involved in enhancing the toxicity of other amines (particularly histamines) [168,169]. Bradycardia, hypotension, paresis of the extremities, and lockjaw are the adverse effects of putrescines found and reported [164,170]. Furthermore, putrescines are able to interreact with nitrites to produce nitrosamines that are carcinogenic [171]. These findings indicate that putrescines should also be risk factors for CVDs.

The level of putrescines in fresh foods seems to be not significant. However, its concentration could be high in spoiled and fermented foods. For example, one of the most common biamines detected in fermented foods is the putrescine. Some food and beverage products rich in putrescines are shown in Table 8.

Gram-negative bacteria (particularly those in the families *Shewanellaceae*, *Pseudomonadaceae*, and *Enterobacteriaceae* that are usually involved in the spoilage of food resources) should be the main microorganisms that can produce putrescines [172]. The genera of *Enterobacteria* including *Shigella*, *Salmonella*, *Proteus*, *Escherichia*, *Klebsiella*, and *Citrobacter* were found to be involved in the synnthesis of considerable quantities of putrescines in foods [173-176]. Some genera of *Enterobacteriaceae* are ornithine decarboxylase phenotypes [177]. Putrescines were also found to be produced by lactic acid bacteria (staphylococci, and mainly lactobacilli) [178-180]. *Oenococcus oeni* (the dominant malolactic fermentation species in wine) is the main fermenting microorganism that produces putrescines though putrescines are also produced during wine fermentation by strains belong to *L. hilgardii* and *L. plantarum* species [162,178,181,182]. It should be noted that the high activity of decarboxylases is found in different bacteria species.

Cadaverine

The cadaverine is another diamine which can be produced in humans, other animals and microorganisms. It can be produced by the decarboxylation of a lysine, which is catalyzed by a lysine decarboxylase. There is another way of producing cadaverines. In this way, cadaverines are produced during the biosynthesis of de novo polyamines [163]. The biological action of cadaverines in humans is not well understood but it might also contribute with the above described polyamines and diamines. Cadaverines were found to be capable of replacing putrescines in some systems (including bacteria) [183].

The ability of cadaverines to cause health problems (including illness in the cardiovascular system) appears to be not as strong as that of tyramines and histamines. It is probable that the adverse effect of dietary cadaverines is involved in enhancing the toxicity of other amines (particularly histamines) [168,169]. Bradycardia, hypotension, paresis of the extremities, and lockjaw are the adverse effects of cadaverines found and reported [164,170]. Furthermore, cadaverines are able to inter-react with nitrites to produce nitrosamines that are carcinogenic [171]. These findings indicate that cadaverines might also increase CVD risks.

Un-used (or extra) cadaverines are degraded to aldehydes via oxidization, which is catalyzed by diamine oxidases [167]. The low activity of diamine oxidases in huams in combination with the high intake of cadaverines would be likely to result in adverse effects.

The level of cadaverines in fresh foods seems to be not significant. However, its concentration could be high in spoiled and fermented foods. Some food and beverage products rich in cadaverines are shown in Table 9.

Table 9. Some food or beverage products rich in cadaverine [161]

Food or Beverage Categories	Cadaverine Content	Food or Beverage Categories	Cadaverine Content
Fermented sausages	37.4 – 38.0 mg/kg	Fermented vegetables	26.0 – 35.4 mg/kg
Other meat products	6.7 – 6.8 mg/kg	Blue cheeses	83.1–121.0 mg/kg
Other ripened meat products	17.2 -17.5 mg/kg	Cheeses	72 – 109 mg/kg
Fish sauces	180 – 182 mg/kg	Acid curd cheeses	628 mg/kg
Other fish and fish products	Up to 1690 mg/kg	Washed rind cheeses	37.4 – 38.0 mg/kg
Fermented fish meats	14 – 17.3 mg/kg	Hard cheeses	47.8 – 83.5 mg/kg

Enterobacteriaceae usually involved in the spoilage of food resources should be the main microorganisms that can produce cadaverines [172]. The genera of *Enterobacteria* including *Shigella*, *Salmonella*, *Proteus*, *Escherichia*, *Klebsiella*, and *Citrobacter* were found to be involved in the synnthesis of considerable quantities of cadaverines in foods [173-176]. Some genera of *Enterobacteriaceae* are lysine decarboxylase phenotypes [177]. Cadaverines were also found to be produced by lactic acid bacteria (staphylococci, and mainly lactobacilli) [178-180]. It should be noted that the high activity of decarboxylases is found in different cadaverine-producing bacteria species.

Phenylethylamine

The phenylethylamine is derived from a phenylalanine by decarboxylation in humans. A monoamine oxidase mediates its metabolism. There are two isomers of monoamine oxidases in humans. One (named monoamine oxidase A) is predominantly found in the placenta, intestine, and stomach [184]. Another one (named monoamine oxidase B) is predominantly found in the brain. A phenylethylamine can also be converted to a noradrenaline (a sympathetic neurotransmitter) by N-methylation catalyzed by a N-methyltransferase. Dopamine-beta-hydroxylase and aldehyde dehydrogenase were also reported to be associated with the metabolism of phenylethylamines [185].

The neuromodulating function of phenylethylamines functionally and structurally links to catecholamines in humans [186]. The indirect sympathomimetic effect (via releasing noradrenalin) of phenylethylamines results in a vasoconstriction as well as transient hypertension in humans. Dietary phenylethylamines were assumed to result in the vasodilatation of the mesenteric vascular bed so that blood flow is elevated at the gastrointestinal level and thus its absorption is facilitated [186]. It was also reported that at the cardiovascular level, phenylethylamines had direct effects (linked to specific receptors) that cause an elevation of the heart rate [187]. These might also be the basis of their adverse effect on the cardiovascular system when they are over-loading.

In addition to hypertension, there are other observed symptoms of toxicity caused by phenylethylamines, for example the dilatation of pupils, headaches, vomiting, perspirations, and so on. After the ingestion of phenylethylamines for 30 minutes to a few hours, it would be able to observe the clinical signs which normally pass away in few hours and the complete recovery time is less than 24 hours. The level of phenylethylamines in fresh foods seems to be trace. However, its concentration could be high in spoiled and fermented foods. Some food and beverage products rich in phenylethylamines are shown in Table 10.

Table 10. Some food or beverage products rich in phenylethylamine [161]

Food or Beverage Categories	Phenylethylamine Content	Food or Beverage Categories	Phenylethylamine Content
Fermented sausages	6.2 – 7.0 mg/kg	Cheeses	3.4 – 5.0 mg/kg
Other meat products	0.5 - 1.9 mg/kg	Blue cheeses	ca. 5.0 mg/kg
Fish sauces	17.2 –20.9 mg/kg	Hard cheeses	ca. 5.0 mg/kg
Other fish and fish products	2.3 - 7.1mg/kg	Beer	0.3- 0.5 mg/kg
Fermented fish meats	0.9 – 3.9 mg/kg		

The activity of tyrosine decarboxylating bacteria during fermentation might be involved in the production of phenylethylamines. This production process of phenylethylamines usually links to the production of tyramines, involving *Staphylococcus*, *Lactobacillus curvatus*, and *Enterococcus* [188-191]. It was also reported that considerable quantities of phenylethylamines were produced by some strains of *S. carnosus* during the fermentation of sausages without the production of tyramines [192-194].

Tryptamine

The tryptamine is derived from a tryptophan by decarboxylation in humans. Its metabolism is mainly mediated by monoamine oxidases (A and B) and is rapid so that its *in vivo* half time is very short.

The neuromodulating function of tryptamines functionally and structurally links to catecholamines in humans [186]. The indirect sympathomimetic effect (via releasing noradrenalin) of tryptamines results in transient hypertension and vasoconstriction in humans. Dietary tryptamines were assumed to induce the vasodilatation of the mesenteric vascular bed so that blood flow is elevated at the gastrointestinal level and thus its absorption is facilitated [186]. It was also reported that at the cardiovascular level, tryptamines had direct effects (linked to specific receptors) which cause an elevation of the heart rate [187]. These might also be the basis of their adverse effect on the cardiovascular system when they are over-loading.

In addition to hypertension, there are other observed symptoms of toxicity caused by tryptamines, for example the dilatation of pupils, headaches, vomiting, perspirations, and so on. After the ingestion of tryptamines for 30 minutes to a few hours, it would be able to observe the clinical signs which normally pass away in few hours and the complete recovery time is less than 24 hours.

The concentration of tryptamines in fresh foods seems to be trace. Nevertheless, the concentration of tryptamines could be high in spoiled and fermented foods. Some food and beverage products rich in tryptamines are shown in Table 11.

Table 11. Some food or beverage products rich in tryptamine [161]

Food or Beverage Categories	Tryptamine Content	Food or Beverage Categories	Tryptamine Content
Fermented sausages	8.3 – 8.5 mg/kg	Fish sauces	88.1 - 93.5 mg/kg
Other meat products	0.2 – 0.9 mg/kg	Cheeses	1 - 46.8 mg/kg
other ripened meat products	0.1 – 0.4 mg/kg	Hard cheeses	1.4 - 45.7 mg/kg
Fermented fish meats	1.0 – 1.2 mg/kg	Acid curd cheeses	134 mg/kg
Other fish and fish products	3.1 - 7.7 mg/kg	Beer	0.2 - 0.7mg/kg

Cyanide

The cyanide at a level less than the lethal dose (0.5-2.9 mg/kg body weight) [195] was identified to be vascularly toxic [196]. The blood levels (0.5 – 1 mg/L) of cyanides resulted in tachycardia [197]. Experiments on goats indicated that an oral daily potassium cyanide intake of 1.2 mg/kg body weight for 5 months caused congestion and hemorrhage in the cerebellum [198]. Studies on intermediate-duration oral exposure (15-364 days) to cyanide compounds suggested a minimum risk CN^- daily level of 0.05 mg/kg body weight [199].

Cyanides exist in such foods as cassavas, sorghums, bamboo shoots, almonds, apples, mangos, and peaches. For example, the reported cyanide levels are 0.001 to 0.45 mg/kg in cereal grains and their products, 0.07 to 0.3 mg/kg in soy protein products, 1 g/kg in cassavas, and 0.1 to 3 g/kg in lima beans [200]. Among cyanides, the hydrogen cyanide is unlikely to be found in well-cooked foods since it is volatile.

References

[1] Tsujita, T., Takaku, T., (2007). Lipolysis induced by segment wall extract from Satsuma mandarin orange (*Citrus unshu* Mark). *J. Nutr. Sci. Vitaminol.* 53(6), 547–551.

[2] Parmar, H.S., Kar, A., (2008). Medicinal values of fruit peels from *Citrus sisensis*, Punica granatum, and Musa paradisiacal with respect to alterations in tissue lipid peroxidation and serum concentration of glucose, insulin, and thyroid hormones. *J. Med. Food* 11(2), 376–381.

[3] Ibrahim, K.E., Couch, M.W., Williams, C.M., Fregly, M.J., Midgley, J.M., (1985). *m*-Octopamine: normal occurrence with *p*-octopamine in mammalian sympathetic nerves. *J. Neurochem.* 44, 1862–1867.

[4] Watson, D.G., Midgley, J.M., Chen, R.N., Huang, W., Bain, G.M., McDonald, N.M., Reid, J.L., McGhee, C.N.J., (1990). Analysis of biogenic amines and their metabolites in biological tissues and fluids by gas chromatography—negative ion chemical ionization mass spectrometry (GC-NICIMS). *J. Pharm. Biomed. Anal.* 8, 899-904.

[5] Wang, R., Wan, L., Li, Q., Liu, X., Huang, Y., (2007). Chemiluminescence of synephrine based on the cerium(IV)–rhodamine B system. *Luminescence* 22, 140–146.

[6] Ibrahim, K.E., Couch, M.W., Williams, C.M., Budd, M.B., Yost, R.A., Midgley, J.M., (1984). Quantitative measurement of octopamines and synephrines in urine using capillary column gas chromatography negative ion chemical ionization mass spectrometry. *Anal. Chem.* 56, 1695–1699.

[7] D'Andrea, G., Terrazzino, S., Fortina, D., Farruggioa, A., Rinaldi, L., Leon, A., (2003). HPLC electrochemical detection of trace amines in human plasma and platelets and expression of mRNA transcripts of trace amine receptors in circulating leukocytes. *Neurosci. Lett.* 346, 89–92.

[8] D'Andrea, G., Granella, F., Leone, M., Perini, F., Farruggio, A., Bussone, G., (2006). Abnormal platelet trace amine profiles in migraine with and without aura. *Cephalalgia* 26, 968–972.

[9] Lasch, F., (1927). Über die Pharmakologie des Sympathols, einer neuen adrenalinähnlichen Substanz. (Zugleich ein Beitrag zur Frage der chemischen

Konstitution und pharmakodynamischen Wirkung). *Naunyn-Schmiedebergs Archiv für Experimentelle Pathologie und Pharmakologie* 124, 231-244.

[10] Lands, A.M., Grant, J.I., (1952). The vasopressor action and toxicity of cyclohexylethylamine derivatives. *J. Pharmacol. Exp. Ther.* 106, 341-345.

[11] Arbo, M.D., Schmitt, G.C., Limberger, M.F., Charão, M.F., Moro, Â.M.,. Ribeiro, G.L., Dallegrave, E., Garcia, S.C., Leal, M.B., Limberger, R.P., (2009). Subchronic toxicity of *Citrus aurantium* L. (Rutaceae) extract and *p*-synephrine in mice. *Regulatory Toxicol. Pharmacol.* 54, 114-117.

[12] Jordan, S., Murty, M., Pilon, K., (2004). Products containing bitter orange or synephrine: suspected cardiovascular adverse reactions. *Can. Med. Assoc. J.* 171, 993–4.

[13] Adams, K.F., Patterson, J.H., Gattis, W.A., O'Connor, C.M., Lee, C.R., Todd, A., Schwartz, T.A., Gheorghiade, M., (2005). Relationship of serum digoxin concentration to mortality and morbidity in women in the digitalis investigation group trial: A retrospective analysis. *J. Am. Coll. Cardiol.* 46, 497–504.

[14] Bui, L.T., Nguyen, D.T., Ambrose, P.J., (2006). Blood pressure and heart rate effects following a single dose of bitter orange. *Ann. Pharmacother.* 40(1), 53–57.

[15] Stohs, S.J., Preuss, H.G., Shara, M., (2011). A review of the receptor-binding properties of p-synephrine as related to its pharmacological effects. *Oxid. Med. Cell. Longev.* 2011, 482973.

[16] Penzak, S.R., Jann, M.W., Cold, J.A., Hon, Y.Y., Desai, H.D., Gurley, B.J., (2001). Seville (sour) orange juice: synephrine content and cardiovascular effects in normotensive adults. *J. Clin. Pharmacol.* 41(10), 1059-63.

[17] Stohs, S.J., Preuss, H.G., Shara, M., (2012). A Review of the Human Clinical Studies Involving *Citrus aurantium* (Bitter Orange) Extract and its Primary Protoalkaloid *p*-Synephrine. *Int. J. Med. Sci.* 9(7), 527-538.

[18] Hansen, D.K., George, N.I., White, G.E., Abdel-Rahman, A., Pellicore, L.S., Fabricant, D., (2013). Cardiovascular Toxicity of *Citrus aurantium* in Exercised Rats. *Cardiovasc. Toxicol.* 13(3), 208-219.

[19] Stewart, I., Newhall, W.F., Edwards, G.J., (1964). The isolation and identification of synephrine in the leaves and fruit of Citrus. *J. Biol. Chem.* 239, 930-932.

[20] Wheaton, T.A., Stewart, I., (1970). The distribution of tyramine, N-methyltyramine, hordenine, octopamine and synephrine in higher plants. *Lloydia* 33, 244-254.

[21] Swinehart, J.A., Stermitz, F.R., (1980). Bishordeninyl terpene alkaloids and other constituents of *Zanthoxylum culantrillo* and *Z. coriaceum*. *Phytochem.* 19, 1219-1223.

[22] Ko, H.C., Chen, K.T., Chen, C.F., Su, J.P., Chen, C.M., Wang, G.J., (2006). Chemical and biological comparisons on *Evodia* with two related species of different locations and conditions. *J. Ethnopharmacol.* 108, 257-263.

[23] Kim, S.P., Moon, E., Nam, S.H., Friedman, M., (2012). Composition of Herba Pogostemonis water extract and protection of infected mice against *Salmonella typhimurium*-induced liver damage and mortality by stimulation of innate immune cells. *J. Agric. Food Chem.* 60, 12122–12130.

[24] Shulgin, A., Shulgin, A., *Tihkal: The Continuation*. Berkeley: Transform Press; 1997; pp. 671. ISBN 0-9630096-9-9.

[25] Bartley, G.E., Breksa III, A.P., Ishida, B.K., (2010). PCR amplification and cloning of tyrosine decarboxylase involved in synephrine biosynthesis in Citrus. *New Biotech.* 27, 308-316.

[26] Wheaton, T.A., Stewart, I., (1969). Biosynthesis of synephrine in citrus. *Phytochem.* 8, 85–92.

[27] Kusu, F., Li, X. D., Takamura, K., (1992). Determination of synephrine and N-methyltyramine in Zhishi and Zhike (immature Citrus fruits) by high-performance liquid chromatography with electrochemical detection. *Chem. Pharm. Bull.*40, 3284-3286.

[28] Pellati, F., Benvenuti, S., Melegari, M., (2005). Enantioselective LC analysis of synephrine in natural products on a protein-based chiral stationary phase. *J. Pharm. Biomed. Anal.* 37, 839-849.

[29] Mattoli, L., Cangi, F., Maidecchi, A., Ghiara, C., Tubaro, M., Traldi, P., (2005). A rapid liquid chromatography electrospray ionization mass spectrometry method for evaluation of synephrine in *Citrus aurantium* L. samples. *J. Agric. Fd. Chem.* 53, 9860–9866.

[30] Avula, B., Upparapalli, S.K., Khan, I.A., (2007). Simultaneous analysis of adrenergic amines and flavonoids in citrus peel jams and fruit juices by liquid chromatography: part 2. *J. AOAC Int.* 90, 633-40.

[31] Kusu, F., Matsumoto, K., Arai, K., Takamura, K., (1996). Determination of synephrine enantiomers in food and conjugated synephrine in urine by high-performance liquid chromatography with electrochemical detection. *Anal. Biochem.* 235, 191-194.

[32] Dragull, K., Breksa, A.P., Cain, B., (2008). Synephrine content of juice from Satsuma Mandarins (*Citrus unshiu* Marcovitch). *J. Ag. Fd. Chem.* 56, 8874-8878.

[33] Vieira, S.M., Theodoro, K.H., Glória, M.B.A., (2007). Profile and levels of bioactive amines in orange juice and orange soft drink. *Food Chem.* 100, 895-903.

[34] Mattoli, L., Cangi, F., Maidecchi, A., Ghiara, C., Tubaro, M., Traldi, P., (2005). A rapid liquid chromatography electrospray ionization mass spectrometry method for evaluation of synephrine in *Citrus aurantium* L. samples. *J. Agric. Fd. Chem.* 53, 9860–9866.

[35] Uckoo, R.M., Jayaprakasha, G.K., Nelson, S.D., Patil, B.S., (2011). Rapid simultaneous determination of amines and organic acids in citrus using high-performance liquid chromatography. *Talanta* 83, 948-54.

[36] Gibson, C.M., Fowler, P.W., (2014). Aromaticity of caffeine, xanthine and the dimethyl xanthines. *Tetrah. Lett.* (55)13, 2078–2081.

[37] Budavari, S., *The Merck Index* (12th ed.). Whitehouse Station, NJ: Merck & Co., Inc; 1996; pp. 1674.

[38] Brittain, H.G., Richard J. Prankerd, R.J., *Profiles of Drug Substances, Excipients and Related Methodology, volume 33: Critical Compilation of* pK_a *Values for Pharmaceutical Substances*. Academic Press; 2007; pp.15. ISBN 0-12-260833-X.

[39] Klosterman, L., *The Facts About Caffeine (Drugs)*. Benchmark Books (NY); 2006; pp.43. ISBN 0-7614-2242-0.

[40] Vallombroso, T., *Organic Chemistry Pearls of Wisdom*. Boston Medical Publishing Corp; 2001; pp.43. ISBN 1-58409-016-2.

[41] Etherton, G.M., Kochar, M.S., (1993). Coffee facts and controversies. *Arch. Fam. Med.* 2(3), 317–322.

[42] Miners, J.O., Birkett, D. J., (1996). The use of caffeine as a metabolic probe for human drug metabolizing enzymes. *Gener. Pharmacol.* (27)2, 245–249.

[43] Miners, J.O., McKinnon, R.A., CYP1A. In: *Metabolic Drug Interactions*, R. H. Levy, K. E. Thummel, W. F. Trager, P. D. Hansten, and M. E. Eichelbaum, Eds.. New York, NY, USA: Lippincott Williams &Wilkins ; 2000; pp. 61–73.

[44] Pardo, P., Garćıa, Y.A., Barral, D., Farré Albaladejo, M., (2007). Caféına: Un nutriente, um f´armaco, o uma droga de abuso. *Adicciones* 19(3), 225–238.

[45] Bispo, M.S., Veloso, M.C.C., Pinheiro, H.L.C., De Oliveira, R.F.S., Reis, J.O.N., Andrade, J.B.D., (2002). Simultaneous determination of caffeine, theobromine, and theophylline by high-performance liquid chromatography. *J. Chromatogr. Sci.* 40(1), 45–48.

[46] Nehlig, A., (1999). Are we dependent upon coffee and caffeine? A review on human and animal data. *Neurosci. Biobehav. Rev.* 23(4), 563–576.

[47] Fredholm, B.B., Bättig, K., Holmén, J., Nehlig, A., Zvartau, E.E., (1999). Actions of caffeine in the brain with special reference to factors that contribute to its widespread use. *Pharmacol. Rev.* 51(1), 83–133.

[48] Arnaud, M.J., Metabolism of caffeine. In: *Caffeine, Coffee and Health*, S. Garatini, Ed.. New York, USA: Raven Press; 1993; pp.43–95.

[49] Temple, N.J., Wilson, T., *Beverages in Nutrition and Health*. Totowa, NJ: Humana Press; 2003; pp.172. ISBN 1-58829-173-1.

[50] Zajac, M.A., Zakrzewski, A.G., Kowal, M.G., Narayan, S., (2003). A Novel Method of Caffeine Synthesis from Uracil. *Synth. Commun.* 33(19), 3291–3297.

[51] Matissek, R., (1997). Evaluation of xanthine derivatives in chocolate: nutritional and chemical aspects. *Europ. Food Res. Technol.* 205(3), 175–84.

[52] Somogyi, LP., (2010). Caffeine Intake by the U.S. Population, prepared for FDA, USA. http://www.fda.gov/downloads/AboutFDA/CentersOffices/OfficeofFoods/CFSAN/CFSANFOIAElectronicReadingRoom/UCM333191.pdf

[53] Viani, R., The composition of coffee, In: *Caffeine, Coffee and Health*, S. Garatini, Ed.. New York, NY, USA: Raven Press;1993; pp. 17–41.

[54] Hicks, M.B., Hsieh, Y. H.P., Bell, L.N., (1996). Tea preparation and its influence on methylxanthine concentration. *Food Res. Intern.* 29(3–4), 325–330.

[55] Bempong, D.K., Houghton, P.J., Steadman, K., (1993). The xanthine content of guarana and its preparations. *Int. J. Pharmacog.* 31(3), 175–181.

[56] Smit, H.J., Gaffan, E.A., Rogers, P.J., (2004). Methylxanthines are the psychopharmacologically active constituents of chocolate. *Psychopharmacol. (Berl.)* 176(3–4), 412–9.

[57] American Psychiatric Association, *Diagnostic and Statistical Manual of Mental Disorders* (4th ed.). American Psychiatric Association; 1994. ISBN 0-89042-062-9.

[58] Holmgren, P., Nordén-Pettersson, L., Ahlner, J., (2004). Caffeine fatalities – four case reports.. *Forens. Sci. Intern.* 139(1), 71–3.

[59] Kamijo, Y., Soma, K., Asari, Y., Ohwada, T., (1999). Severe rhabdomyolysis following massive ingestion of oolong tea: caffeine intoxication with coexisting hyponatremia. *Vet. Hum. Toxicol.* 41(6), 381-3.

[60] Verkhratsky, A., (2005). Physiology and pathophysiology of the calcium store in the endoplasmic reticulum of neurons. *Physiol. Rev.* 85(1), 201–79.

[61] *Mrvos, R.M., Reilly, P.E., Dean, B.S., Krenzelok, E.P., (1989). Massive caffeine ingestion resulting in death. Vet. Hum. Toxicol. 31(6), 571-2.*

[62] *Walsh, I., Wasserman, G.S., Mestad, P., Lanman, R.C., (1987). Near-fatal caffeine intoxication treated with peritoneal dialysis. Pediatr. Emerg. Care 3(4), 244-9.*

[63] *Kerrigan, S., Lindsey, T., (2005). Fatal caffeine overdose: two case reports. Forens. Sci. Int. 153(1), 67-9.*

[64] Peters, J.M., (1967). Factors Affecting Caffeine Toxicity: A Review of the Literature. *J. Clin. Pharmacol. J. New Drugs* 7(7), 131–141.

[65] LaCroix, A.Z., Mead, L.A., Liang, K.Y., Thomas, C.B., Pearson, T.A., (1986). Coffee consumption and the incidence of coronary heart disease. *N. Engl. J. Med.* 315, 977-82.

[66] Panagiotakos, D.B., Pitsavos, C., Chrysohoou, C., Kokkinos, P., Toutouzas, P., Stefanadis, C., (2003). The J-shaped effect of coffee consumption on the risk of developing acute coronary syndromes: The CARDIO 2000 case-control study. *J. Nutr.* 133, 3228-32.

[67] Happonen, P., Voutilainen, S., Salonen, J.T., (2004). Coffee drinking is dose-dependently related to the risk of acute coronary events in middle-aged men. *J. Nutr.* 134, 2381-6.

[68] Grobbe, D.E., Rimm, E.B., Giovannucci, E., Colditz, G., Stampfer, M., Willett, W., (1990). Coffee, Caffeine and cardiovascular disease in men. *N. Engl. J. Med.* 323, 1026-32.

[69] Kleemola, P., Jousilahti, P., Pietinen, P., Vartiainen, E., Tuomilehto, J., (2000). Coffee consumption and the risk of coronary heart disease and death. *Arch. Intern. Med.* 160, 3393-400.

[70] Lane, J.D., Pieper, C.F., Phillips-Bute, B.G., Bryant, J.E., Kuhn, C.M., (2002). Caffeine affects cardiovascular and neuroendocrine activation at work and home. *Psychosom. Med.* 64, 595–603.

[71] Basheer, R., Strecker, R.E., Thakkar, M.M., McCarley, R.W., (2004). Adenosine and sleep-wake regulation. *Progr. Neurobiol.* 73(6), 379-396.

[72] Lovallo, W.R., Wilson, M.F., Vincent, A.S., Sung, B.H., McKey, B.S., Whitsett, T.L., (2004). Blood pressure response to caffeine shows incomplete tolerance after short-term regular consumption. *Hypertens.* 43, 760–5.

[73] Savoca, M.R., Conner, D., Evans, C.D., Wilson, M.E., Harshfield, G.A., Ludwig, D.A., (2004). The Association of caffeinated beverages with blood pressure in adolescents. *Arch. Pediatr. Adolesc. Med.* 158, 473-7.

[74] Amaresh, N., Mullaicharam, A.R., El-Khider, M.A., (2011). Chemistry and pharmacology of caffeine in different types of tea leaves. *Int. J. Nutr. Pharmacol. Neurol. Dis.* 1, 110-5.

[75] Pilli, R., Naidu, M., Pingali, U.R., Takallapally, R.R., (2012). Study of cardiovascular effects of caffeine in healthy human subjects, with special reference to pulse wave velocity using photoplethysmography. *Int. J. Nutr. Pharmacol. Neurol. Dis.* 2, 243-50.

[76] Vlachopoulos, C., Hirata, K., O'Rourke, M.F., (2003). Effect of caffeine on aortic elastic properties and wave reflection. *J. Hypertens.* 21, 563-70.

[77] Papaioannou, T.G., Karatzi, K., Karatzis, E., Papamichael, C., Lekakis, J.P., (2005). Acute effects of caffeine on arterial stiffness, wave reflections, and central aortic pressures. *Am. J. Hypertens.* 18, 129-36.

[78] Mahmud, A., Feeley, J., (2001). Acute effect of caffeine on arterial stiffness and aortic pressure waveform. *Hypertens.* 38, 227-31.

[79] Vlachopoulos, C., Panagiotakos, D., Ioakeimidis, N., Dima, I., Stefanadis, C., (2005). Chronic coffee consumption has a detrimental effect on aortic stiffness and wave reflections. *Am. J. Clin. Nutr.* 81, 1307-12.

[80] Vlachopoulos, C., Hirata, K., Stefanadis, C., Toutouzas, P., O'Rourke, M.F., (2003). Caffeine increases aortic stiffness in hypertensive patients. *Am. J. Hypertens.* 16, 63-6.

[81] Ilbäck, N.G., Siller, M., Stalhandske, T., (2007). Evaluation of cardiovascular effects of caffeine using telemetric monitoring in the conscious rats. *Food Chem. Toxicol.* 45(5), 834-842.

[82] Mahmud, A., Feely, J., (2001). Acute effect of caffeine on arterial stiffness and aortic pressure waveform. *Hypertens.* 38, 227-231.

[83] Howden, R., Hanlon, P.R., Petranka, J.G., Kleeberger, S., Bucher, J., Dunnick, J., Nyska, A., Murphy, E., (2005). Ephedrine plus caffeine causes age-dependent cardiovascular responses in Fischer 344 rats. *Am. J. Physiol. Heart Circ. Physiol.* 288(5), H2219-2224.

[84] Mehta, A., Jain, A.C., Mehta, M.C., Billie, M., (1997). Caffeine and cardiac arrhythmias. An experimental study in dogs with review of literature. *Acta Cardiol.* 52(3), 273-283.

[85] Conen, D., Chiuve, S.E., Everett, B.M., Zhang, S.M., Buring, J.E., Albert, C.M., (2010). Caffeine consumption and incident atrial fibrillation in women. *Am. J. Clin. Nutr.* 92, 509–514.

[86] Pelchovitz, D.J., Goldberger, J.J., (2011). Caffeine and cardiac arrhythmias: A review of the evidence. *Am. J. Med.* 124, 284-9.

[87] Sutphin, G.L., Bishop, E., Yanos, M.E., Moller, R.M., Kaeberlein, M., (2012). Caffeine extends life span, improves healthspan, and delays age-associated pathology in *Caenorhabditis elegans*. *Longev. Healthsp.* 1, 9.

[88] Ammon, H.P., Bieck, P.R., Mandalaz, D., Verspohl, E.J., (1983). Adaptation of blood pressure to continuous heavy coffee drinking in young volunteers. A double-blind crossover study. *Br. J. Clin. Pharmacol.* 15, 701-6.

[89] Robertson, D., Wade, D., Workman, R., Woolsey, R.L., Oates, J.A., (1981). Tolerance to the humoral and hemodynamic effects of caffeine in man. *J. Clin. Invest.* 67, 1111-7.

[90] Robertson, D., Hollister, A.S., Kincaid, D., Workman, R., Goldberg, M.R., Tung, C.S., Smith, B., (1984). Caffeine and hypertension. *Am. J. Med.* 77, 54-60.

[91] Ding, M., Bhupathiraju, S.N., Satija, A., van Dam, R.M., Hu, F.B., (2014). Long-Term Coffee Consumption and Risk of Cardiovascular Disease: A Systematic Review and a Dose–Response Meta-Analysis of Prospective Cohort Studies. *Circulation* 129, 643-659.

[92] Philips, S.R., Rozdilsky, B., Boulton, A.A., (1978). Evidence for the presence of m-tyramine, p-tyramine, tryptamine, and phenylethylamine in the rat brain and several areas of the human brain. *Biol. Psych.* 13(1), 51–57.

[93] Lindemann, L., Hoener, M.C., (2005). A renaissance in trace amines inspired by a novel GPCR family. *Trends Pharmacol. Sci.* 26(5), 274–281.

[94] Broadley, K.J., (2010). The vascular effects of trace amines and amphetamines. *Pharmacol. Ther.* 125(3), 363–375.

[95] Liberles, B., (2006). A second class of chemosensory receptors in the olfactory epithelium. *Nature* 441(7103), 645–650.

[96] Navarro, H.A., Gilmour, B.P., Lewin, A.H., (2006). A Rapid Functional Assay for the Human Trace Amine-Associated Receptor 1 Based on the Mobilization of Internal Calcium. *J. Biomol. Screen* 11(6), 668–693.

[97] Xie, Z., Westmoreland, S.V., Miller, G.M., (2008). Modulation of monoamine transporters by common biogenic amines via trace amine-associated receptor 1 and monoamine autoreceptors in human embryonic kidney 293 cells and brain synaptosomes. *J. Pharm.* 441(2), 629–640.

[98] Rao, T.S.S., Yeragani, V.K., (2009). Hypertensive crisis and cheese Indian *J. Psych.* 51(1), 65–66.

[99] Mitchell, E.S., Antidepressants. In: Drugs, the Straight Facts, edited by David J. Triggle. Chelsea House Publishers; 2004.

[100] Stahl, S.M., Felker, A., (2008). Monoamine oxidase inhibitors: a modern guide to an unrequited class of antidepressants. *Cns. Spectrums.* 13(10), 855–870.

[101] Jacob, L.H., Carron, D.B., (1987). Atrial fibrillation precipitated by tyramine containing foods. *Brit. Heart J.* 57, 205-6.

[102] Tiller, J.W.G., Maguire, K.P., Davies, B.M., Dowling, J.T., Tung, L.H., Rand, M.J., (1990). Tyramine-induced cardiac arrhythmias. *Hum. Psychopharmacol: Clin. Exper.* 5, 313–321.

[103] Bieck, P.R., Antonin, K.H., (1988). Oral tyramine pressor tests the safety of monoamine oxidase inhibitor drugs: comparison of brofaromine and tranylcypromine in healthy subjects. *J. Clin. Psychopharmacol.* 8, 237–245.

[104] Da Prada, M., Zurcher, G., Wuthrich, I., (1988). On tyramine, food, beverages: the reversible MAO inhibitor moclobemide. *J. Neur. Transm.* 26, 31–36.

[105] Numata, A., Miyauchi, Y., Ono, N., Fishbein, M.C., Mandel, W.J., Lin, S.F., Weiss, J.N., Chen, P.S., Karagueuzian, H.S., (2012). Spontaneous atrial fibrillation initiated by tyramine in canine atria with increased sympathetic nerve sprouting. *J. Cardiovasc. Electrophysiol.* 23(4), 415-22.

[106] Smith, T. A., (1977). Phenethylamines and related compounds in plants. *Phytochem.* 16, 9-18.

[107] Walker, S.E., Shulman, K.I., Tailor, S.A., Gardner, D., (1996). Tyramine content of previously restricted foods in monoamine oxidase inhibitor diets. *J. Clin. Psychopharmacol.* 16(5), 383-8.

[108] Paulsen, P., Grossgut, R., Bauer, F., Rauscher-Gabernig, E., (2012). Estimates of maximum tolerable levels of tyramine content in foods in Austria. *J. Food Nutr. Res.* 51(1), 52–59.

[109] De Backer, D., Biston, P., Devriendt, J., Madl, C., Chochrad, D., Aldecoa, C., Brasseur, A., Defrance, P., Gottignies, P., Vincent, J.L., (2010). Comparison of Dopamine and Norepinephrine in the Treatment of Shock. *New Engl. J. Med.* 362(9), 779–789.

[110] Bryant, B.J., Knights, K.M., *Pharmacology for Health Professionals* (2nd ed.). Australia: Elsevier; 2009; pp.192. ISBN 978-0-7295-3929-6.

[111] Karthik, S., Lisbon, A., (2006). Low-dose dopamine in the intensive care unit. *Semin. Dial.* 19(6), 465–71.

[112] WHO Model List of Essential Medicines, *World Health Organization*; 2013. October 2013. Available at: http://www.who.int/medicines/publications/essentialmedicines/en/index.html

[113] Geiger, B.M., Frank, L.E., Caldera-Siu, A.D., Stiles, L., Pothos, E.N., (2007). Deficiency of central dopamine in multiple obesity models. *Appetite* 49(1), 293-293.

[114] Zhang, M.Z., Yao, B., Wang, S., Fan, X., Wu, G., Yang, H., Yin, H., Yang, S., Harris, R.C., (2011). Intrarenal dopamine deficiency leads to hypertension and decreased longevity in mice. *J. Clin. Invest.* 121(7), 2845–2854.

[115] Bruckner, J.B., Hess, W., Schmidt, D., Schneider, E., Schweichel, E., (1977). Dopamine effects on circulation and myocardial oxygen supply. *Proc. Roy. Soc. Med.* 70(Suppl.2), 43-47.

[116] Sulzer, D., Zecca, L., (2000). Intraneuronal dopamine-quinone synthesis: a review. *Neurotox. Res.* 1(3), 181–95.

[117] Goyoaga, C., Burbano, C., Cuadrado, C., Varela, A., Guillamón, E., Pedrosa, M.M., Muzquiz, M., (2008). Content and distribution of vicine, convicine and l -DOPA during germination and seedling growth of two Vicia faba L. varieties. *Eur. Food Res. Technol.* 227, 1537-42.

[118] Kanazawa, K., Sakakibara, H., (2000). High content of dopamine, a strong antioxidant, in Cavendish banana. *J. Agr. Food Chem.* 48(3), 844-8.

[119] Kulma, A., Szopa, J., (2007). Catecholamines are active compounds in plants. *Plant Sci.* 172(3), 433–440.

[120] Van Alstyne, K.L., Nelson, A.V., Vyvyan, J.R., Cancilla, D.A., (2006). Dopamine functions as an antiherbivore defense in the temperate green alga *Ulvaria obscure*. *Oecologia* 148(2), 304–11.

[121] Wichers, H.J., Visser, J.F., Huizing, H.J., Pras, N., (1993). Occurrence of L-DOPA and dopamine in plants and cell cultures of *Mucuna pruriens* and effects of 2, 4-d and NaCl on these compounds. *Plant Cell, Tiss. Org. Cult.* 33(3), 259–264.

[122] Longo, R., Castellani, A., Sberze, P., Tibolla, M., (1974). Distribution of l-dopa and related amino acids in Vicia. *Phytochem.* 13(1), 167–171.

[123] Ingle, P.K., (2003). L-DOPA bearing plants. *Nat. Prod. Rad.* 2, 126–133.

[124] Young, S.N., (2007). How to increase serotonin in the human brain without drugs. *Rev. Psychiatr. Neurosci.* 32(6), 394–99.

[125] Berger, M., Gray, J.A., Roth, B.L., (2009). The expanded biology of serotonin. *Annu. Rev. Med.* 60, 355–66.

[126] Côté, F., Thévenot, E., Fligny, C., Fromes, Y., Darmon, M., Ripoche, M.A., Bayard, E., Hanoun, N., Saurini, F., Lechat, P., Dandolo, L., Hamon, M., Mallet, J., Vodjdani, G., (2003). Disruption of the nonneuronal tph1 gene demonstrates the importance of peripheral serotonin in cardiac function. *Proc. Natl. Acad. Sci. U.S.A.* 100(23), 13525–30.

[127] Turner, E.H., Loftis, J.M., Blackwell, A.D., (2006). Serotonin a la carte: supplementation with the serotonin precursor 5-hydroxytryptophan. *Pharmacol. Therapeutics.* 109(3), 325-38.

[128] Baskin, S.I., *Principles of cardiac toxicology*. Boca Raton: CRC Press; 1991.

[129] Nakatani, Y., Sato-Suzuki, I., Tsujino, N., Nakasato, A., Seki, Y., Fumoto, M., Arita, H., (2008). Augmented brain 5-HT crosses the blood-brain barrier through the 5-HT transporter in rat. *Eur. J. Neurosci.* 27(9), 2466-72.

[130] Savelieva, K.V., Zhao, S., Pogorelov, V.M., Rajan, I., Yang, Q., Cullinan, E., Lanthorn, T.H., (2008). Bartolomucci, Alessandro, ed. Genetic disruption of both tryptophan hydroxylase genes dramatically reduces serotonin and affects behavior in models sensitive to antidepressants. *PLoS ONE* 3(10), e3301.

[131] Feldman, J.M., Lee, E.M., (1985). Serotonin content of foods: effect on urinary excretion of 5-hydroxyindoleacetic acid. *Am. J. Clin. Nutr.* 42(4), 639–43.

[132] Guillén-Casla, V., Rosales-Conrado, N., León-González, M.E., Pérez-Arribas, L.V., Polo-Díez, L.M., (2012). Determination of serotonin and its precursors in chocolate samples by capillary liquid chromatography with mass spectrometry detection. *J. Chromatogr. A* 1232, 158–65.

[133] USDA Agricultural Research Service, USDA national nutrient database for standard reference. Updated on September 29, 2008. Accessed 23 October 2008. URL: http://www.nal.usda.gov/fnic/foodcomp/search/. 2008. http://www.nal.usda.gov/fnic/ foodcomp/ search/. 2008.

[134] Monograph, (2006). L-tryptophan. *Altern. Med. Rev.* 11:52–56. Accessed 11 December 2008. URL: http://web.ebscohost.com.libproxy.uthscsa.edu/ehost/results?vid=2&hid=117&sid=d83bc99c-3f42-4802-832f-a31552298d7f%40sessionmgr103&bquery=(JN+%22Alternative+Medicine+Review%22+and+DT+20060301)&bdata=JmRiPWF3aCZ0eXBlPTEmc2l0ZT1laG9zdC1saXZl.

[135] Harper, A.E., Yoshimura, N.N., (1993). Protein quality, amino acid balance, utilization, and evaluation of diets containing amino acids as therapeutic agents. *Nutr.* 9, 460–9.

[136] Rambali, B., Van Andel, I., Schenk, E., Wolterink, G., van de Werken, G., Stevenson, H., Vleeming W., The contribution of cocoa additive to cigarette smoking addiction. RIVM report 650270002/2002. The National Institute for Public Health and the Environment (Netherlands); 2002.

[137] FAO/WHO/UNU., Energy and Protein Requirements. Report of a joint FAO/WHO/UNU Expert Consultation. Technical Report Series no. 724, World Health Organization, Geneva, Switzerland; 1985.

[138] FAO/WHO., Energy and Protein Requirements. Technical Report Series no. 522, World Health Organization, Geneva, Switzerland; 1973.

[139] Dougherty, D.M., Marsh, D.M., Mathias, C.W., Dawes, M.A., Bradley, D.M., Morgan, C.J., Badawy, A.A., (2007). The effects of alcohol on laboratory-measured impulsivity after L-Tryptophan depletion or loading. *Psychopharmacol. (Berl)* 193, 137–50.

[140] Badawy, A.A., Morgan, C.J., Lovett, J.W., Bradley, D.M., Thomas, R., (1995). Decrease in circulating tryptophan availability to the brain after acute ethanol consumption by normal volunteers: Implications for alcohol-induced aggressive behaviour and depression. *Pharmacopsych.* 28, 93–7.

[141] Marieb, E., *Human anatomy & physiology*. San Francisco: Benjamin Cummings; 2001; pp.414. ISBN 0-8053-4989-8.

[142] Di Giuseppe, M., Sergienko, A.V., Saleh, B.E.A., *Nelson Biology 12*. Toronto: Thomson Canada; 2003; pp.473. ISBN 0-17-625987-2.

[143] Cabanié, M., Godfraind, T., (1988). The role of histamine in the cardiovascular system. *Drugs Exp. Clin. Res.* 14(2-3), 141-7.

[144] Bartholomew, B.A., Berry, P.R., Rodhouse, J.C., Gilbert, R.J., Murray, C.K., (1987). Scombrotoxic fish poisoning in Britain: features of over 250 suspected incidents from 1976 to 1986. *Epidemiol. Infect.* 99, 775-782.

[145] Li, H., Burkhardt, C., Heinrich, U.R., Brausch, I., Xia, N., Förstermann, U., (2003). Histamine upregulates gene expression of endothelial nitric oxide synthase in human vascular endothelial cells. *Circulation* 107(18), 2348–2354.

[146] Liao, W., Rudling, M., Angelin, B., (1997). Novel effects of histamine on lipoprotein metabolism: suppression of hepatic low density lipoprotein receptor expression and reduction of plasma high density lipoprotein cholesterol in the rat. *Endocrinol.* 138(5), 1863–1870.

[147] Lindstedt, K.A., Mäyränpää, M.I., Kovanen, P.T., (2007). Mast cells in vulnerable atherosclerotic plaques—a view to a kill. *J. Cell. Molec. Med.* 11(4), 739–758.

[148] Zdravkovic, V., Pantovic, S., Rosic, G., Tomic-Lucic, A., Zdravkovic, N., Colic, M., Obradovic, Z., Rosic, M., (2011). Histamine Blood Concentration in Ischemic Heart Disease Patients. *J. Biomed. Biotechnol.* 2011, Article ID 315709, 8 pages. http://dx.doi.org/10.1155/2011/315709

[149] Coultate, T.D., FOOD: The Chemistry of Its Components, 2nd edition. Royal Society of Chemistry, Cambridge; 1989; pp.287-288.

[150] Pontiroli, A.E., Pozza, G., (1978). HISTAMINE STIMULATES PROLACTIN RELEASE IN NORMAL MEN. *Acta Endocrinol.* 88, 23-28.

[151] Özogul, F., Özogul, Y., (2006). Biogenic amine content and biogenic amine quality indices of sardines (Sardina pilchardus) stored in modified atmosphere packaging and vacuum packaging. *Food Chem.* 99, 574–578.

[152] Kanki, M., Yoda, T., Ishibashi, M., Tsukamoto, T., (2004). Photobacterium phosphoreum caused a histamine fish poisoning incident. *Int. J. Food Microbiol.* 92, 1, 79–87.

[153] Emborg, J., Dalgaard, P., Ahrens, P., (2006). Morganella psychrotolerans sp. nov., a histamine producing bacterium isolated from various seafoods. *Int. J. System. Evolut. Microbiol.* 56, 2473- 2479.

[154] Dalgaard, P., Emborg, J., Kjolby, A., Sorensen, N., Ballin, N., Histamine and biogenic amines - formation and importance in seafood. In: Improving seafood products for the consumer. Borrensen T, ed. Cambridge, UK: Woodhead Publishing Ltd.; 2008.

[155] Vanderslice, P., Copeland, W.C., Robertus, J.D., (1986). Cloning and nucleotide sequence of wild type and a mutant histidine decarboxylase from Lactobacillus 30a. *J. Biol. Chem.* 261, 15186-15191.

[156] Spano, G., Russo, P., Lonvaud-Funel, A., Lucas, P., Alexandre, H., Grandvalet, C., Coton, E., Coton, M., Barnavon, L., Bach, B., Rattray, F., Bunte, A., Magni, C., Alvarez, M., Fernandez, M., Lopez, P., Barcelo, P., Corbi, A., Lolkema, J.S., (2010). Risk assessment of biogenic amines in fermented food. *Europ. J. Clin. Nutr.* 64, 95-100.

[157] Beutling, D.M., Biogene Amine in der Ernährung. Wien - Berlin - New York: Springer; 1996.

[158] Kimura, B., Konagaya, Y., Fujii, T., (2001). Histamine formation by Tetragenococcus muriaticus, a halophilic lactic acid bacterium isolated from fish sausae. *Int. J. Food Microbiol.* 70, 71-77.

[159] Lucas, P.M., Wolken, W.A.M., Claisse, O., Lolkema, J.S., Lonvaud-Funel, A., (2005). Histamine-producing pathway encoded on an unstable plasmid in Lactobacillus hilgardii 0006. *Appl. Environ. Microbiol.* 71, 1417-1424.

[160] Costantini, A., Vaudano, E., Prete, V.D., Danei, M., Garcia-Moruno, E., (2009). Biogenic amine production by contaminating bacteria found in starter preparations used in winemaking. *J. Agric. Food Chem.* 57, 22, 10664-10669.

[161] EFSA Panel on Biological Hazards (BIOHAZ), (2011). Scientific Opinion on risk based control of biogenic amine formation in fermented foods. *EFSA J.* 9(10), 2393. [93 pp.] Doi:10.2903/j.efsa.2011.2393.

[162] Lucas, P.M., Blancato, V.S., Claisse, O., Magni, C., Lolkema, J.S., Lonvaud-Funel, A., (2007). Agmatine deiminase pathway genes in Lactobacillus brevis are linked to the tyrosine decarboxylation operon in a putative acid resistance locus. *Microbiol.* 153, 2221-2230.

[163] Bardocz, S., (1995). Polyamines in food and their consequences for food quality and human health. *Trends Food Sci. Technol.* 6(10), 341-346.

[164] Halász, A., Baráth. Á., Toxicity of biogenic amines – the present knowledge. In Food Science and technology COST 917 Biogenically active amines in food, Vol VI. Luxembourg: EC Publication; 2002; pp 131-141.

[165] Löser, C., Eisel, A., Harms, D., Fölsch, U., (1999). Dietary polyamines are essential luminal growth factors for small intestinal and colonic mucosal growth and development. *Gut* 44, 1, 12–16.

[166] Farriol, M., Segovia-Silvestre, T., Castellanos, J.M., Venereo, Y., Orta, X., (2001). Role of putrescine in cell proliferation in a colon carcinoma cell line. *Nutr.* 17(11-12), 934-938.

[167] Askar, A., Treptow, H., Biogene Amine in Lebensmitteln: Vorkommen, Bedeutung und Bestimmung, Ulmer, Stuttgart; 1986.

[168] Chu, C.H., Bjeldanes, L.F., (1981). Effect of diamines, polyamines and tuna fish extracts on the binding of histamine to mucin in vitro. *J. Food Sci.* 47(1), 79-80, 88.

[169] Hui, J.Y., Taylor, S.L., (1985). Inhibition of in vivo histamine metabolism in rats by foodborne and pharmacologic inhibitors of diamine oxidase, histamine N-methyltransferase, and monoamine oxidase. *Toxicol. Appl. Pharmacol.* 81(2), 241-249.

[170] Shalaby, A.R., (1996). Significance of biogenic amines to food safety and human health. *Food Res. Int.* 29(7), 675-690.

[171] Nebelin, E., Pillai, S., Lund, E., Thomsen, J., (1980). On the formation of N-nitrosopyrrolidine from potential precursors and nitrite. *IARC Scient. Public.* 31, 183-193.

[172] Lopez-Caballero, M.E., Sanchez-Fernandez, J.A., Moral, A., (2001). Growth and metabolic activity of Shewanella putrefaciens maintained under different CO2 and O2 concentrations. *Int. J. Food Microbiol.* 64(3), 277-287.

[173] Paleologos, E.K., Savvaidis, I.N., Kontominas, M.G., (2004). Biogenic amines formation and its relation to microbiological and sensory attributes in ice-stored whole, gutted and filleted Mediterranean Sea bass (Dicentrarchus labrax). *Food Microbiol.* 21(5), 549-557.

[174] Kim, M.K., Mah, J.H., Hwang, H.J., (2009). Biogenic amine formation and bacterial contribution in fish, squid and shellfish. *Food Chem.* 116, 87–95.

[175] Rezaei, M., Montazeri, N., Langrudi, H.E., Mokhayer, B., Parviz, M., Nazarinia, A., (2007). The biogenic amines and bacterial changes of farmed rainbow trout (Oncorhynchus mykiss) stored in ice. *Food Chem.* 103, 150–154.

[176] Chytiri, S., Paleologos, E., Savvaidis, I., Kontominas, M.G., (2004). Relation of biogenic amines with microbial and sensory changes of whole and filleted freshwaterrainbow trout (Oncorhynchus mykiss) stored on ice. *J. Food Prot.* 67(5), 960–965.

[177] Moeller, V., (1954). Distribution of amino acid decarboxylase in Enterobacteriaceae. *Acta Pathol. Microbiol. Scand.* 35(3), 259-277.

[178] Arena, M.E., Manca de Nadra, M.C., (2001). Biogenic amine production by Lactobacillus. *J. Appl. Microbiol.* 90, 158-162.

[179] Beneduce, L., Romano, A., Capozzi, V., Lucas, P., Barnavon, L., Bach, B., Vuchot, P., Grieco, F., Spano, G., (2010). Biogenic amine in wines. *Ann. Microbiol.* 60, 573-578.

[180] Coton, E., Mulder, N., Coton, M., Pochet, S., Trip, H., Lolkema, J.S., (2010). Origin of the putrescineproducing ability of the coagulase-negative bacterium Staphylococcus epidermidis 2015B. *Appl. Environ. Microbiol.* 76, 5570-5576.

[181] Nannelli, F., Claisse, O., Gindreau, E., de Revel, G., Lonvaud-Funel, A., Lucas, P.M., (2008). Determination of lactic acid bacteria producing biogenic amines in wine by quantitative PCR methods. *Lett. Appl. Microbiol.* 47, 594–599.

[182] Marcobal, A., de las Rivas, B., Moreno-Arribas, M.V., Muñoz, R., (2004). Identification of the ornithine decarboxylase gene in the putrescine producer Oenococcus oeni BIFI-83. *FEMS Microbiol. Lett.* 239, 213-220.

[183] Hölttä, E., Pohjanpelto, P., (1983). Polyamine starvation causes accumulation of cadaverine and its derivatives in a polyamine-dependet strain of Chinese-hamster ovary cells. *Biochem. J.* 210, 945- 948.

[184] Suzuki, O., Katsumata, Y., Oya, M., (1981). Oxidation of β-Phenylethylamine by Both Types of Monoamine Oxidase: Examination of Enzymes in Brain and Liver Mitochondria of Eight Species. *J. Neurochem.* 36(3), 1298–301.

[185] Sabelli, H.C., Javaid, J.I., (1995). Phenylethylamine modulation of affect: therapeutic and diagnostic implications. *J. Neuropsych. Clin. Neurosci.* 7(1), 6–14.

[186] Broadley, K.H., (2010). The vascular effects of trace amines and amphetamines. *Pharmacol. Therap.* 125, 363-375.

[187] Frascarelli, S., Gghelardoni, S., Chiellini, G., Vardiu, R., Ronca-Testoni, S., Scalan, T.S., Grandy, D.K., Zucchi, R., (2008). Cardiac effects of trace amines: pharmacological characterization of trace aminesassociated receptors. *European J. Pharmacol.* 587, 1-3, 231-236.

[188] Bover-Cid, S., Hugas, M., Izquierdo-Pulido, M., Vidal-Carou, M.C., (2000). Amino acid-decarboxylase activity of bacteria isolated from fermented pork sausages. *Int. J. Food Microbiol.* 66(3), 185–189.

[189] Bover-Cid, S., Hernández-Jover, T., Miguélez-Arrizado, M.J., Vidal-Carou, M.C., (2003). Contribution of contaminant enterobacteria and lactic acid bacteria to biogenic amine accumulation in spontaneous fermentation of pork sausages. *Europ. Food Res. Technol.* 216(6), 477-482.

[190] Moreno-Arribas, M.V., Lonvaud-Funel, A., (2001). Purification and characterization of tyrosine decarboxylase of Lactobacillus brevis IOEB 9809 isolated from wine. *FEMS Microbiol. Lett.* 195, 103–107.

[191] Suzzi, G., Gardini, F., (2003). Biogenic amines in dry fermented sausages: a review. *Int. J. Food Microbiol.* 88, 1, 41-54.

[192] Ansorena, D., Montel, M.C., Rokka, M., Talon, R., Enrola, S., Rizzo, A., Raemaekers, M., Demeyer, D., (2002). Analysis of biogenic amines in northern and southern European sausages and role of flora in amine production. *Meat Sci.* 61, 141-147.

[193] De las Rivas, B., Ruiz-Capillas, C., Carrascosa, A.V., Curiel, J.A., Jiménez-Colmenero, F., Muñoz, R., (2008). Biogenic amine production by Gram-positive bacteria isolated from Spanish dry cured "chorizo" sausage treated with high pressure and kept in chilled storage. *Meat Sci.* 80, 2,272-277.

[194] Latorre-Moratalla, M.L., Bover-Cid, S., Talon, R., Aymerich, T., Garriga, M., Zanardi, E., Ianieri, A., Fraqueza, M.J., Elias, M., Drosinos, E.H., Laukovà, A., Vidal-Carou, M.C., (2009). Distribution of aminogenic activity among potential autochthonous starter cultures for dry fermented sausages. *J. Food Prot.* 73, 3, 524-528.

[195] U.S. Environmental Protection Agency (USEPA), Health effects criteria document for cyanide. Washington, D.C.: Office of Drinking Water; 1985.

[196] Branton, P.J., McAdam, K.G., Winter, D.B., Liu, C., Duke, M.G., Proctor, C.J., (2011). Reduction of aldehydes and hydrogen cyanide yields in mainstream cigarette smoke using an amine functionalised ion exchange resin. *Chem. Centr. J.* 5, 15.

[197] Linden, C.H., Lovejoy, F.H., Poisoning and drug overdose. In: AS Francos, E Braunwald, KJ Isselbacher, editor, Harrison's principles of internal medicine. New York: McGraw-Hill Health Professions Division; 1998.

[198] Soto-Blanco, B., Maiorka, P.C., Górniak, S.L., (2002). Neuropathologic study of long term cyanide administration to goats. *Food Chem. Toxicol.* 40(Iss.11), 1693–8.

[199] Taylor, J., Toxicological Profile for Cyanide (Update). Darby, P.A.: DIANE Publishing; 2010; pp.322.

[200] Honig, D.H., Hockridge, M.E., Gould, R.M., Rackis, J.J., (1983). Determination of cyanide in soybeans and soybean products. *J. Agr. Food Chem.* 31, 272-5.

Chapter 8

Overconsumption of Uric Acid-Increasing Diets

The uric acid consists of nitrogen, oxygen, carbon, and hydrogen. It is an aromatic compound. Its formula is $C_5H_4N_4O_3$ and the diagram of its heterocyclic structure is shown in Figure 18.

The acidity of an uric acid is weak, and its pKa_1 or pKa_2 is 5.4 or 10.3, respectively [1]. Therefore, it is diprotic and has the pKa_1 < that of carbonic acid. Under the condition of a biological pH, it becomes an acid urate ion that is singly charged. This compound and its alkali metal salts have a quite low solubility in water. These properties may be the basis of their unique biological effects.

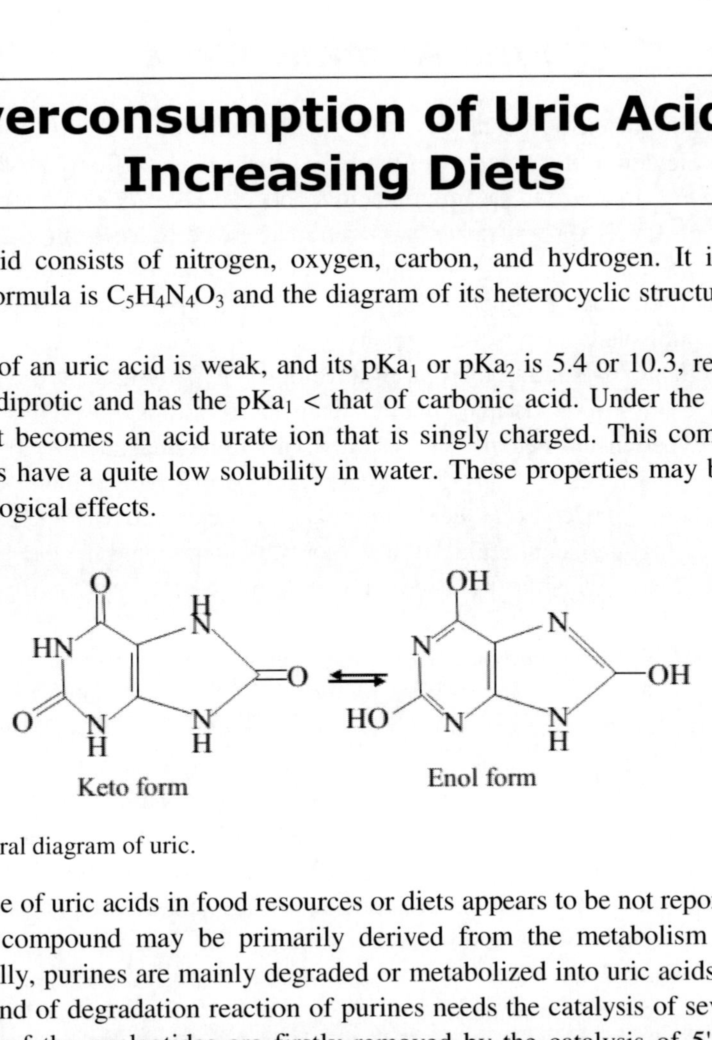

Figure 18. Structural diagram of uric.

The presence of uric acids in food resources or diets appears to be not reported in the past literature. This compound may be primarily derived from the metabolism of purines in humans. Generally, purines are mainly degraded or metabolized into uric acids in the liver in humans. This kind of degradation reaction of purines needs the catalysis of several enzymes. The phosphates of the nucleotides are firstly removed by the catalysis of 5'-nucleotidases. Second, through the catalysis of the adenosine deaminases or nucleosidases, adenosines or nucleosides are hydrolyzed and deaminated, respectively, to become hypoxanthines. Then, xanthines are formed via the oxidation of hypoxanthines. The formed xanthines are ultimately converted to uric acids via the catalysis of xanthine oxidases. The guanosine is also a purine nucleoside, which can be firstly degraded to produce a guanine. Guanine deaminases catalyze the deamination of guanines to produce xanthines. Uric acids are finally formed by the conversion of xanthines via the way similar to that just described above. The ultimate acceptor of electrons is oxygen throughout the period of degrading both purines. Generally, more than 70% of urates are excreted via renals [2]. And also, there are various forms of excretion of uric acids from the body in different animals [3].

The upper end of the normal range of uric acid levels in the human blood was reported to be 7 mg/dL (412 μmol/L) for men or 6 mg/dL (360 μmol/L) for women [4]. The normal value range of uric acids in the human blood was stated to be 2.5 to 7.0 mg/dL in men and 1.5 to 6.0 mg/dL in women [5].

Uric Acid and CVDs

An increase in nucleic acid intake is a risk factor for hyper-uric acid concentrations in the blood [6]. The elevation of uric acids in the blood may increase the risk of CVDs [7,8], for example, a 1 mg/dL increase in serum uric acid levels caused a 26% increase in mortality [9]. The elevation of levels of uric acids was reported to correlate with the increase in the prevalence of hypertension [10,11]. The uric acid concentration in serum was reported to be an independent predictor of hypertension (glomerular hypertension) and hyperinsulinemia [7,8]. Another published paper stated that hyperuricemia was consistently proved to be an independent factor for predicting the risk of developing hypertension by several studies [12]. The increased serum uric acids may also result in the development of renal arteriosclerosis that can make hypertension become salt-sensitive and renal-dependent [13]. The mechanism of uric acids, having the effects described above, may be involved in their potential ability to decrease endothelial nitric oxide concentrations. A vasoreactive hypertension might be initiated by the high concentration of uric acids, which could further become kidney-dependent [5]. This conclusion might be supported by the fact that the hyperuricemia was found to be independently associated with renal dysfunction [14-16] and microalbuminuria [17] and that there was a correlation between the reduced function of kidneys and the elevated concentrations of uric acids in individuals who were healthy and normotensive [18]. Furthermore, the elevated morbidity of hypertension was found to be positively linked to the high concentrations of uric acids in the plasma in adults [19,20]. Particularly, it was reported that diastolic hypertension was predicted by the concentrations of uric acids in plasma though systolic hypertension was not [21,22]. Nevertheless, it should be noted that this kind of correlation might be reduced by patient's ages [23] and it was not observed in patients who were elder [21, 24-26]. The weakening relationship between uric acids and hypertension with ages has few possible explanations. For example, salt sensitive hypertension that is irreversible can result from small renal vessels damaged by increased uric acid levels and continue with the reduced concentrations of uric acids [27]. Moreover, the hyperuricemia may just be a weaker predictor of hypertension developing in the elder individuals than other pathophysiological factors for example the reduced compliance of arteria [28]. This might be supported by the following finding that weight gains, systolic hypertension, hypertriglyceridemia, and hyperinsulinemia were prevented by the administration of drugs reducing uric acid levels [5]. Study in babies born low weights also indicated that hypertension is associated with hyperuricemia [29]. It seems that babies born low weights are more likely to develop hypertension that is linked to elevated concentrations of uric acids in their later life [30]. There was another investigation involving ten Caucasians who had essential hypertension (aged 35 - 59 years old) that also indicated a positive association of hypertension with the decreased number of nephrons [31]. Therefore, it was assumed that babies born low weights have smaller number of nephrons and hypertension risks are greater [32]. It should be particularly noted that the increased level of uric acids in the mother was found to be a major risk factor for babies born low weights [33,34]. All those published papers mentioned above appear to indicate the positive association of the development of hypertension with the high concentrations of uric acids though the elevated level of uric acids might possibly result from the mere consequence of diseases.

It seems that the hyperuricemia is independently associated with the elevated risk of a coronary heart disease (CHD) or linked-events with the absence of other risk factors for a CHD and especially a predictor of increased risk of CHD mortality in females. The CHD is an illness that is defined as a decreased blood injection to the muscle of the heart, usually because of narrowed coronary arteries and atherosclerotic lesions. For example, each increase in 1 mg/dL of uric acids in a patient with a CHD was found to be linked to a 12% elevation of mortality of CHDs, which was the result of a meta-analysis of a prospective cohort study [35]. The hyperuricemia was found to be associated with ca. 70% elevation of CHD risks in females though no association was found in males [5]. This finding was consistent with the result of a meta-analysis of the past published results which indicated that the hyperuricemia was positively linked to the significantly elevated risk of CHDs in both females and males [10]. The authors did not find that the prediction of CHDs by independently using serum uric acids was significant. Nevertheless, the authors did show that the odds ratio of increased serum uric acids was larger than 1 after the adjustment of other possible coordinators and risk factors that had been established. Further study is required for understanding the mechanisms in relation to the association of the hyperuricemia with an increased risk of CHDs in females and it is believed that this kind of study is very worthwhile.

It seems that the hyperuricemia is also associated with the increased risk of other CVDs. For example, in the Apolipoprotein Mortality Risk Study, the authors investigated into the potential of elevated uric acids as the risk factors for strokes, congestive heart failures, and acute myocardial infarctions [36]. The authors finally concluded that the elevated risk of both ischemic and hemorrhagic strokes was linked to the elevated concentrations of uric acids. Another study concluded that the hyperuricemia is a cofactor of increasing the risk of developing CVDs, such as strokes [35]. It has been reported that, in the United States, ca. 1/18 deaths are caused by strokes which are in the third rank of the leading factor for deaths [5]. Furthermore, it was reported that strokes occurred in about 795,000 Americans every year, which was equivalent to about 1 stroke per 40 seconds [37]. Meta-analysis and large systematic reviews that analyzed the association of the hyperuricemia with the morbidity and mortality of strokes can be found in the past literature [11]. This review collected a total of 16 prospective cohort studies involving more than 230,000 individuals who had CVDs. The results of the analysis in this paper indicated that the hyperuricemia greatly increased the mortality and morbidity of strokes, as compared to the normal levels of uric acids in controls. And also, the authors concluded that there was still a significant association of the hyperuricemia with strokes after the adjustment of other established factors for increasing stroke risks.

There are also many studies indicated a positive association of the hyperuricemia with metabolic syndromes that is linked to CVDs. A metabolic syndrome may be defined as an abnormal condition associated with a prothrombotic and proinflammatory state, insulin resistance, dyslipidemia, abdominal obesity, and hypertension [38,39]. The characteristics of diagnosing the metabolic syndrome are usually as the combination of three or more of the following risk measurements: fasting glucose concentrations (>110 mg/dL), blood pressure (>130/>85 mmHg), HDLC (<50 mg/dL for females, <40 mg/dL for males), triglycerides (>150 mg/dL), and waist circumference (>88 cm for females, and >102 cm for males) [5]. The dramatic increase in the occurrence of metabolic syndromes in the United States was reported and its prevalence in 2000 was ca. 27% [40]. The risk of inducing CVDs is higher in individuals with a metabolic syndrome, compared with those without it [41]. It was reported by several authors that the metabolic syndrome developed in industrialized countries worldwide is linked to the hyperuricemia [42-44]. From the 1920s to the 1970s, the plasma concentrations of uric acids increased from the average of 3.5 mg/dL to 6.5 mg/dL in the general population [45,46]. The inhibition of nitric oxide synthases by uric acids might be the mechanism of developing metabolic syndromes [47,48]. There is one investigation supporting this theory which indicated the development of features of metabolic syndromes including elevated insulin resistance, hypertriglyceridemia, hypercholesterolemia, and hypertension in knockout mice lacking nitric oxide synthases [49].

The hyperuricemia is likely to cause both vascular and interstitial inflammation that may be responsible for developing CVDs. It appear to be certain that the crystals of uric acids in the blood greatly result in the dysfunction of the vascular system and inflammation in humans though the published opinion on the effect of soluble uric acids may be conflicting [50]. It is generally believed that uric acids with their concentrations > 6.8 mg/dL in the blood can crystallize into monosodium urate [5].

Diets Increasing Uric Acid

There are considerable amounts of purine bases in some foods. The purines exist in food resources in forms of free molecules and included in RNA or DNA. Free purines primarily include guanine, adenine, xanthine, and hypoxanthine. There was a published paper that reported the determined content of free purines and total purines in 31 processed and fresh food products [51]. The authors employed perchloric acids in hydrolyzing the conjugated purines in nucleic acids for 1 h at 100°C and liberating them for quantification. They found that the highest sources of purine bases were meat products. They also concluded that the highest total purine sources were organ meats, but there were equivalent quantities of the uricogenic bases (hypoxanthine + adenine) in all the meat samples. They further stated that among all samples analyzed, breads and dairy products had the lowest purine content while mushrooms had some purine bases content as great as that of some meats. Another study analyzed the concentrations of total and free purine bases (guanine, adenine, xanthine and hypoxanthine) in cooked (boiled and broiled) and fresh haddock fillets, beef livers, and beef steaks [52]. They found that cooking modified the uricogenicity of meat products since the high concentration of free xanthines and hypoxanthines was found in the cooking juices of steaks.

Many foods contain significant amounts of nucleic acids. Food materials containing 1500-10000 mg/kg nucleic acids include pheasants, quails, grouses, rabbits/hares, venisons, organ meats (kidneys, hearts, sweetbreads, livers, pâtés, terrines, liver sausages), fish roes (cod roes, caviars, taramasalatas), scallops, herrings, mackerels, trouts, crayfishes, lobsters, some small fishes eaten whole or processed (such as anchovies, sardines, sprats, whitebaits, and their processed products) [53].

The nucleic acids are usually digested in the small intestine. The enzymes nucleases (RNAse and DNAse) from the pancreas catalyze the degradation of the nucleic acids to nucleotides. Then, alkaline phosphatases catalyze the conversion of the nucleotides to nucleosides. The sodium-coupled active transport takes up the nucleosides (including uricogenic purines).

It also seems that an elevation of fructoses is associated with the rising incidence of the hyperuricemia as well as hypertension. For example, it was reported that ATP was found to be quickly depleted and the concentrations of uric acids in the blood was increased by the increased ingestion of fructoses [54]. Animal study also found that the ingestion of fructoses induced the development of metabolic syndromes, including higher body weights, hypertension, higher triglycerides, and increased insulins, in rats without drugs that could reduce uric acids [55]. It was also reported that the elevated ingestion of fructoses was possibly responsible for the elevation of uric acids in industrialized countries [56,57]. More reports can be found in the past literature, which stated a positively direct association of the ingestion of fructoses with the hyperuricemia [58,59] and may subsequently cause hypertension [60,61] and metabolic syndromes [62,63]. Perhaps, the over consumption of table sugars and the high-fructose corn syrup in the modern human diets caused the over-ingestion of fructoses. This might largely contribute to the trends of rising hypertension as well as uric acid levels in the blood.

References

[1] McCrudden, F.H., *Uric Acid.* BiblioBazaar; 2008. ISBN-10: 0-554-61991-1; ISBN-13: 978-0-554-61991-0

[2] Lipkowitz, M.S., (2012). Regulation of uric acid excretion by the kidney. *Curr. Rheumatol. Rep.* 14(2), 179-88.

[3] Nelson, D.L., Cox, M.M., Lehninger, A.L., *Lehninger's Principles of Biochemistry* (5 ed.). Macmillan; 2008. ISBN 978-0716771081.

[4] Chizyński, K., Rózycka, M., (2005). Hyperuricemia. *Pol. Merkur. Lekarski* (in Polish) 19(113), 693–6.

[5] Jin, M., Yang, F., Yang, I., Yin, Y., Luo, J.J., Wang, H., Yang, X.F., (2012). Uric Acid, Hyperuricemia and Vascular Diseases. *Front. Biosci.* 17, 656–669.

[6] Clifford, A.J., Riumallo, J.A., Young, V.R., Scrimshaw, N.S., (1976). Effect of oral purines on serum and urinary uric acid of normal, hyperuricemic and gouty humans. *J. Nutr.* 106, 428-434.

[7] Ford, E.S., Li, C., Cook, S., Choi, H.K., (2007). Serum concentrations of uric acid and the metabolic syndrome among US children and adolescents. *Circulation* 115, 2526–32.

[8] Forman, J.P., Choi, H., Curhan, G.C., (2007). Plasma uric acid level and risk for incident hypertension among men. *J. Am. Soc. Nephrol.* 18, 287–92.

[9] Alderman, M., Aiyer, K.J.V., (2004). Uric acid: Role in cardiovascular disease and effects of Losartan. *Curr. Med. Res. Opin.* 20(3), 369-79.

[10] Wheeler, J.G., Juzwishin, K.D., Eiriksdottir, G., Gudnason, V., Danesh, J., (2005). Serum uric acid and coronary heart disease in 9,458 incident cases and 155,084 controls: prospective study and meta-analysis. *PLoS Med.* 2, e76.

[11] Kim, S.Y., Guevara, J.P., Kim, K.M., Choi, H.K., Heitjan, D.F., Albert, D.A., (2009). Hyperuricemia and risk of stroke: a systematic review and meta-analysis. *Arthr. Rheum.* 61, 885–92.

[12] Heinig, M., Johnson, R.J., (2006). Role of uric acid in hypertension, renal disease, and metabolic syndrome. *Clevel. Clin. J. Med.* 73, 1059–64.

[13] Johnson, R.J., Herrera-Acosta, J., Schreiner, G.F., Rodriguez-Iturbe, B., (2002). Subtle acquired renal injury as a mechanism of salt-sensitive hypertension. *N. Engl. J. Med.* 346, 913–23.

[14] Tomita, M., Mizuno, S., Yamanaka, H., Hosoda, Y., Sakuma, K., Matuoka, Y., Odaka, M., Yamaguchi, M., Yosida, H., Morisawa, H., Murayama, T., (2000). Does hyperuricemia affect mortality? A prospective cohort study of Japanese male workers. *J. Epidemiol.* 10, 403–9.

[15] Iseki, K., Oshiro, S., Tozawa, M., Iseki, C., Ikemiya, Y., Takishita, S., (2001). Significance of hyperuricemia on the early detection of renal failure in a cohort of screened subjects. *Hypertens. Res.* 24, 691– 7.

[16] Iseki, K., Ikemiya, Y., Inoue, T., Iseki, C., Kinjo, K., Takishita, S., (2004). Significance of hyperuricemia as a risk factor for developing ESRD in a screened cohort. *Am. J. Kidney Dis.* 44, 642–50.

[17] Lee, J.E., Kim, Y.G., Choi, Y.H., Huh, W., Kim, D.J., Oh, H.Y., (2006). Serum uric acid is associated with microalbuminuria in prehypertension. *Hypertens.* 47, 962–7.

[18] Bellomo, G., Venanzi, S., Verdura, C., Saronio, P., Esposito, A., Timio, M., (2010). Association of uric acid with change in kidney function in healthy normotensive individuals. *Am. J. Kidney Dis.* 56, 264– 72.

[19] Chu, N.F., Wang, D.J., Liou, S.H., Shieh, S.M., (2000). Relationship between hyperuricemia and other cardiovascular disease risk factors among adult males in Taiwan. *Eur. J. Epidemiol.* 16, 13–7.

[20] Cigolini, M., Targher, G., Tonoli, M., Manara, F., Muggeo, M., De Sandre, G., (1995). Hyperuricaemia: relationships to body fat distribution and other components of the insulin resistance syndrome in 38-year-old healthy men and women. *Int. J. Obes. Relat. Metab. Disord.* 19, 92–6.

[21] Leite, M.L., (2011). Uric acid and fibrinogen: age-modulated relationships with blood pressure components. *J. Hum. Hypertens.* 25(8), 476-83.

[22] Yeh, C.J., Pan, W.H., Jong, Y.S., Kuo, Y.Y., Lo, C.H., (2001). Incidence and predictors of isolated systolic hypertension and isolated diastolic hypertension in Taiwan. *J. Formos. Med. Assoc.* 100, 668– 75.

[23] Brand, F.N., McGee, D.L., Kannel, W.B., Stokes, J., Castelli, W.P., (1985). Hyperuricemia as a risk factor of coronary heart disease: The Framingham Study. *Am. J. Epidemiol.* 121, 11–8.

[24] Forman, J.P., Choi, H., Curhan, G.C., (2007). Plasma uric acid level and risk for incident hypertension among men. *J. Am. Soc. Nephrol.* 18, 287–92.

[25] Lu, Z., Dong, B., Wu, H., Chen, T., Zhang, Y., Wu, J., Xiao, H., (2009). Serum uric acid level in primary hypertension among Chinese nonagenarians/centenarians. *J. Hum. Hypertens.* 23, 113–21.

[26] Kosugi, T., Nakagawa, T., Kamath, D., Johnson, R.J., (2009). Uric acid and hypertension: an age-related relationship? *J. Hum. Hypertens.* 23, 75–6.

[27] Watanabe, S., Kang, D.H., Feng, L., Nakagawa, T., Kanellis, J., Lan, H., Mazzali, M., Johnson, R.J., (2002). Uric acid, hominoid evolution, and the pathogenesis of salt-sensitivity. *Hypertension.* 40, 355–60.

[28] Blacher, J., Safar, M., (2002). Specific aspects of high blood pressure in the elderly. *J. Renin. Angiotensin Aldosterone Syst.* 3(Suppl 1), S10–5.

[29] Barker, D.J., Osmond, C., Golding, J., Kuh, D., Wadsworth, M.E., (1989). Growth in utero, blood pressure in childhood and adult life, and mortality from cardiovascular disease. *Bmj.* 298, 564–7.

[30] Feig, D.I., Nakagawa, T., Karumanchi, S.A., Oliver, W.J., Kang, D.H., Finch, J., Johnson, R.J., (2004). Hypothesis: Uric acid, nephron number, and the pathogenesis of essential hypertension. *Kidney Int.* 66, 281–7.

[31] Keller, G., Zimmer, G., Mall, G., Ritz, E., Amann, K., (2003). Nephron number in patients with primary hypertension. *N. Engl. J. Med.* 348, 101–8.

[32] Brenner, B.M., Garcia, D.L., Anderson, S., (1988). Glomeruli and blood pressure. Less of one, more the other? *Am. J. Hypertens.* 1, 335–47.

[33] *Roberts, J.M., Bodnar, L.M., Lain, K.Y., Hubel, C.A., Markovic, N., Ness, R.B., Powers, R.W., (2005). Uric acid is as important as proteinuria in identifying fetal risk in women with gestational hypertension. Hypertens.* 46, 1263–*1269.*

[34] *Chang, F.M., Chow, S.N., Huang, H.C., Hsieh, F.J., Chen, H.Y., Lee, T.Y., Ouyang, P.C., Chen, Y.P., (1987). The placental transfer and concentration difference in maternal and neonatal serum uric acid at parturition: comparison of normal pregnancy and gestosis. Biol. Res. Pregnancy Perinatol.* 35, 35–*39.*

[35] Kim, S.Y., Guevara, J.P., Kim, K.M., Choi, H.K., Heitjan, D.F., Albert, D.A., (2010). Hyperuricemia and coronary heart disease: a systematic review and meta-analysis. Arthr. Care Res. 62, 170–80.

[36] Holme, I., Aastveit, A.H., Hammar, N., Jungner, I., Walldius, G., (2009). Uric acid and risk of myocardial infarction, stroke and congestive heart failure in 417,734 men and women in the Apolipoprotein Mortality Risk Study (AMORIS). *J. Intern. Med.* 266(6), 558–70.

[37] Lloyd-Jones, D., Adams, R.J., Brown, T.M., Carnethon, M., Dai, S., De Simone, G., Ferguson, T.B., Ford, E., Furie, K., Gillespie, C., Go, A., Greenlund, K., Haase, N., Hailpern, S., Ho, P.M., Howard, V., Kissela, B., Kittner, S., Lackland, D., Lisabeth, L., Marelli, A., McDermott, M.M., Meigs, J., Mozaffarian, D., Mussolino, M, Nichol, G., Roger, V.L., Rosamond, W., Sacco, R., Sorlie, P., Roger, V.L., Thom, T., Wasserthiel-Smoller, S., Wong, N.D., Wylie-Rosett, J., (2010). Heart disease and stroke statistics--2010 update: a report from the American Heart Association. *Circulation* 121, e46–e215.

[38] Eckel, R.H., Grundy, S.M., Zimmet, P.Z., (2005). The metabolic syndrome. *Lancet.* 365, 1415–28.

[39] Grundy, S.M., Cleeman, J.I., Daniels, S.R., Donato, K.A., Eckel, R.H., Franklin, B.A., Gordon, D.J., Krauss, R.M., Savage, P.J., Smith, S.C., Spertus, J.A., Costa, F., (2005). Diagnosis and Management of the Metabolic Syndrome: An American Heart Association/National Heart, Lung, and Blood Institute Scientific Statement. *Circulation*112, 2735-2752.

[40] Ford, E.S., Giles, W.H., Mokdad, A.H., (2004). Increasing prevalence of the metabolic syndrome among U.S. Adults. *Diabetes Care* 27, 2444–9.

[41] Malik, S., Wong, N.D., Franklin, S.S., Kamath, T.V., (2004). L'Italien GJ, Pio JR, Williams GR. Impact of the metabolic syndrome on mortality from coronary heart disease, cardiovascular disease, and all causes in United States adults. *Circulation* 110, 1245–50.

[42] Onat, A., Uyarel, H., Hergenc, G., Karabulut, A., Albayrak, S., Sari, I., Yazici, M., Keles, I., (2006). Serum uric acid is a determinant of metabolic syndrome in a population-based study. *Am. J. Hypertens.* 19, 1055–62.

[43] Choi, H.K., Ford, E.S., (2007). Prevalence of the metabolic syndrome in individuals with hyperuricemia. *Am. J. Med.* 120, 442–7.

[44] Yoo, T.W., Sung, K.C., Shin, H.S., Kim, B.J., Kim, B.S., Kang, J.H., Lee, M.H., Park, J.R., Kim, H., Rhee, E.J., Lee, W.Y., Kim, S.W., Ryu, S.H., Keum, D.G., (2005). Relationship between serum uric acid concentration and insulin resistance and metabolic syndrome. *Circ. J.* 69, 928–33.

[45] Freedman, D.S., Williamson, D.F., Gunter, E.W., Byers, T., (1995). Relation of serum uric acid to mortality and ischemic heart disease. The NHANES I Epidemiologic Follow-up Study. *Am. J. Epidemiol.* 141, 637–44.

[46] Hall, A.P., Barry, P.E., Dawber, T.R., McNamara, P.M., (1967). Epidemiology of gout and hyperuricemia. A long-term population study. *Am. J. Med.* 42, 27–37.

[47] Khosla, U.M., Zharikov, S., Finch, J.L., Nakagawa, T., Roncal, C., Mu, W., Krotova, K., Block, E.R., Prabhakar, S., Johnson, R.J., (2005). Hyperuricemia induces endothelial dysfunction. *Kidney Int.* 67, 1739–42.

[48] Mazzali, M., Hughes, J., Kim, Y.G., Jefferson, J.A., Kang, D.H., Gordon, K.L., Lan, H.Y., Kivlighn, S., Johnson, R.J., (2001). Elevated uric acid increases blood pressure in the rat by a novel crystal-independent mechanism. *Hypertens.* 38, 1101–6.

[49] Cook, S., Hugli, O., Egli, M., Vollenweider, P., Burcelin, R., Nicod, P., Thorens, B., Scherrer, U., (2003). Clustering of cardiovascular risk factors mimicking the human metabolic syndrome X in eNOS null mice. *Swiss. Med. Wkly.* 133, 360–3.

[50] Yajima, N., Takahashi, M., Morimoto, H., Shiba, Y., Takahashi, Y., Masumoto, J., Ise, H., Sagara, J., Nakayama, J., Taniguchi, S., Ikeda, U., (2008). Critical role of bone marrow apoptosis-associated speck-like protein, an inflammasome adaptor molecule, in neointimal formation after vascular injury in mice. *Circulation* 117, 3079–87.

[51] Brulé, D., Sarwar, G., Savoiet, L., (1988). Purine content of selected canadian food products. *Food Comp. Anal.* 1(2), 130–138.

[52] Brulé, D., Sarwar, G., Savoie, L., (1989). Effect of Methods of Cooking on Free and Total Purine Bases in Meat and Fish. *Can. Inst. Food Sci. Technol. J.* 22(3), 248–251.

[53] Grahame, R., Simmonds, A.H., Carrey, E., Gout. London: Class Publishing (London), Ltd.; 2003. ISBN ISBN 9781859591895

[54] Emmerson, B.T., (1974). Effect of oral fructose on urate production. *Ann. Rheum. Dis.* 33, 276–80.

[55] Nakagawa, T., Hu, H., Zharikov, S., Tuttle, K.R., Short, R.A., Glushakova, O., Ouyang, X., Feig, D.I., Block, E.R., Herrera-Acosta, J., Patel, J.M., Johnson, R.J., (2006). A causal role for uric acid in fructose-induced metabolic syndrome. *Am. J. Physiol. Renal. Physiol.* 290, F625–31.

[56] Johnson, R.J., Segal, M.S., Sautin, Y., Nakagawa, T., Feig, D.I., Kang, D.H., Gersch, M.S., Benner, S., Sanchez-Lozada, L.G., (2007). Potential role of sugar (fructose) in the epidemic of hypertension, obesity and the metabolic syndrome, diabetes, kidney disease, and cardiovascular disease. *Am. J. Clin. Nutr.* 86, 899–906.

[57] Havel, P.J., (2005). Dietary fructose: implications for dysregulation of energy homeostasis and lipid/ carbohydrate metabolism. *Nutr. Rev.* 63, 133–57.

[58] Gao, X., Qi, L., Qiao, N., Choi, H.K., Curhan, G., Tucker, K.L., Ascherio, A., (2007). Intake of added sugar and sugar-sweetened drink and serum uric acid concentration in US men and women. *Hypertens.* 50, 306–12.

[59] Choi, J.W., Ford, E.S., Gao, X., Choi, H.K., (2008). Sugar-sweetened soft drinks, diet soft drinks, and serum uric acid level: the Third National Health and Nutrition Examination Survey. *Arthr. Rheum.* 59, 109–16.

[60] Brown, C.M., Dulloo, A.G., Yepuri, G., Montani, J.P., (2008). Fructose ingestion acutely elevates blood pressure in healthy young humans. *Am. J. Physiol. Regul. Integr. Comp. Physiol.* 294, R730–7.

[61] Schulze, M.B., Manson, J.E., Ludwig, D.S., Colditz, G.A., Stampfer, M.J., Willett, W.C., Hu, F.B., (2004). Sugarsweetened beverages, weight gain, and incidence of type 2 diabetes in young and middle-aged women. *JAMA.* 292, 927–34.

[62] Ludwig, D.S., Peterson, K.E., Gortmaker, S.L., (2001). Relation between consumption of sugar-sweetened drinks and childhood obesity: a prospective, observational analysis. *Lancet.* 357, 505–8.

[63] Segal, M.S., Gollub, E., Johnson, R.J., (2007). Is the fructose index more relevant with regards to cardiovascular disease than the glycemic index? *Eur. J. Nutr.* 46, 406–17.

Chapter 9

Overconsumption of Trimethylamine N-Oxide-Increasing Diets

The formula of the trimethylamine *N*-oxide is $(CH_3)_3NO$. Its structural diagram is shown in Figure 19. This organic compound is a colorless solid that is usually dihydrated. Its solubility in water is good. This compound is found in animals [1] and derived from the oxidation of a trimethylamine that is produced from the conversion of a choline. In humans, it is normally excreted with urine.

It seems that no information related to the absorption of trimethylamine *N*-oxides by the human body can be found in the literature. Since this compound has a small molecular weight and good solubility in water, and exists in some kinds of food resources, its absorption rate through the mucosa of the human intestine and its effect on health might not be ignorable. Therefore, it is very worth carrying out experiment on the absorption rate of trimethylamine *N*-oxides by the human body.

There are two important food components that contain cholines. One is phospholipids, such as lecithin (phosphatidylcholine). Another one is L-carnitines. Generally, phospholipids participate in forming micells whith bile, fatty acids and other fatty materials during the digestion and absorption of foods. However, there are still some phospholipids that are not absorbed. The unabsorped phospholipids can be degraded to release cholines. Once choline-containing compounds are in the cecum and large bowels, they may be utilized as energy sources by intestinal microbiota (gut flora). Therefore, in the intestine, the conversion of cholines into trimethylamines results from the action of gut flora (e.g. species of *Acinetobacter*, Clostridia, Proteus, Shigella). The cholines in L-carnitines can also be converted to trimethylamines by the action of gut flora. It was reported that L-carnitines can be metabolized by multiple bacterial strains [2], and some distinct species within the genus *Clostridium* were found to be capable of metabolizing cholines though some others were not [3]. Then, the trimethylamines (gases) are taken up by the blood and circulated. Once absorbed, the trimethylamines (gases) are quickly converted to trimethylamine *N*-oxides, catalyzed by hepatic flavin mono-oxygenases. The flavin mono-oxygenase 3 should be the main enzyme that is involved in the oxidation of trimethylamines, since fish malodor syndromes because of accumulating trimethylamines were observed in the individuals with mutations in this enzyme [4].

One critical question is what effect of trimethylamine *N*-oxides on human health, particularly the cardiovascular system, would be. Furthermore, what are the cholin-containing sources? Are the cholin-containing compounds present in common food resources? What is the level of cholin-containing compounds in the food materials or resources that contain it?

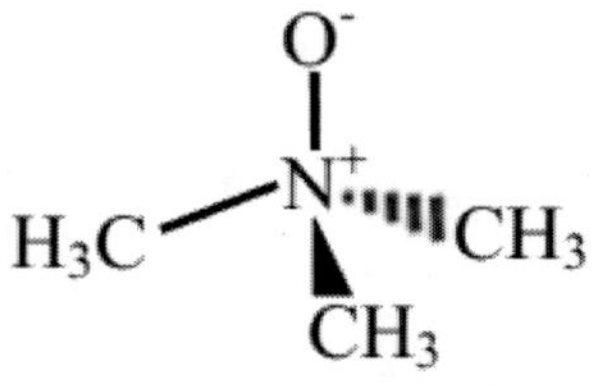

Figure 19. Structural diagram of trimethylamine *N*-oxide.

Trimethylamine N-oxide and CVDs

The increased plasma levels of trimethylamine N-oxides are dose-dependently associated with the presence of CVDs. For example, the results of investigations indicated that the increased concentrations of trimethylamine N-oxides in the blood were linked to an elevated risk of inducing the major adverse incidence of CVDs [5].

Trimethylamine N-Oxide and Atherosclerosis

The rapid metabolism of the absorbed trimethylamine gases by the hepatic flavin monooxygenase family of enzymes results in trimethylamine N-oxides which is positively associated with atherosclerosis [5-7]. It seems that the involvement of trimethylamine N-oxides in developing atherosclerosis may be partly due to its capability of increasing the accumulation of cholesterols within macrophages (maybe induction of scavenger receptors for example SRA1 or CD36), both of which are associated with the uptake of lipoproteins that were modified [6].

Trimethylamine N-Oxide and Hypertension

A recently published paper reported the result of a study on the effect of carnitine-derived trimethylamine N-oxides on blood pressure in rats [8]. The authors designed the following experimental procedures: implanting telemetric transmitters in Sprague-Dawley rats (Twelve-week-old); continuously recording the diastolic blood pressure, the systolic blood pressure, and the heart rate for 7 days before and 14 days during subcutaneous infusions, which was driven by osmotic minipumps, of Ang II + trimethylamine N-oxides, low-dose Ang II, trimethylamine N-oxides, or saline (controls); and estimating the level of trimethylamine N-oxides in plasma by employing a liquid chromatography coupled with a triple-quadrupole mass spectrometry. They found that trimethylamine N-oxides prolonged the hypertensive effect of the Ang II though it did not affect the blood pressure in normotensive rats. It should be noted that the results just mentioned above were caused by the 10 times lower level of trimethylamine N-oxides in the experimental rats than that reported in humans stated by them in the published paper.

Trimethylamine N-Oxide and Blood Lipid Profile

The alteration of metabolism of cholesterols in the wall of arteria, in the liver, and in the intestine may be associated with trimethylamine N-oxides. For example, it was reported that trimethylamine N-oxides elevated the accumulation of macrophage cholesterols and this was found to depend on the action of microbiota via elevating the expression of two scavenger receptors that are proatherogenic (i.e. cluster of scavenger receptor A and differentiation 36) on the surface of cells [6,9,10]. The reverse transportation of cholesterols is inhibited and the sterol metabolism is altered by trimethylamine N-oxides [6].

General Mechanism of Association of Trimethylamine N-Oxide with CVDs

The mechanism of association of trimethylamine N-oxides with CVDs may involve: 1, the pathway of the trimethylamine N-oxide production; 2, the action of trimethylamine N-oxides. For the first possible mechanism, for example, a strong effect of a genetic locus, which contains the flavin monooxygenase (for converting trimethylamines to trimethylamine N-oxides) gene cluster on chromosome 1, on atherosclerosis was reported [6]. For the second possible mechanism, the authors also found that trimethylamine N-oxides enhanced the cell surface expression of two macrophage scavenger receptors associated with atherosclerosis, CD36 and SRA1. Furthermore, trimethylamine N-oxides inhibit the reverse cholesterol transport (RCT), and change a major pathway for removing cholesterols from the body, the pathway of the bile acid synthesis (such as significantly decreasing the expression of the key enzymes, cytochrome P450, family 7, subfamily a, polypeptide 1 (Cyp7a1) and cytochrome P450, family 27, subfamily a, and polypeptide 1 (Cyp27a1), for bile acid synthesis in the liver) [7].

Dietary Sources and Control of Trimethylamine N-Oxide

It seems that the diet-derived production of trimethylamine N-oxides needs the combination of two factors. They include the action of gut bacteria and choline-containing food components that remain in the food residue after the digestion and absorption of nutrients.

The efficiency of converting phosphatidylcholines or L-carnitines to trimethylamine gases and then trimethylamine N-oxides in the blood is dependent on intestinal microbes (*Prevotella* being more powerful than *Bacteroides*). The inhibition of those gut bacteria that can convert choline-containing compounds into trimethylamine gases would certainly reduce the level of trimethylamine N-oxides in the blood. For example, the ingestion of antibiotics should be effective on the reduction of trimethylamine N-oxides in the blood. The suppression of these microbes by antibiotics may greatly decrease plasma trimethylamine N-oxide levels and, subsequently, reduce the risk of atherosclerosis. However, the intake of antibiotics for long term might result in other health problems.

The choline is an essential nutrient for growing and maintaining a human life [11]. Normally, the human body is able to produce this compound and this can meet most of body's requirements. The ingestion of some cholines in daily diets still be necessary since the lack of them could cause neurologic disorders, altered metabolic pathways of one-carbon methyl donors, and a fatty liver [12-15]. The ingestion of 425 mg/day and 550 mg/day of cholines has been suggested to be the Adequate Intake for adult females and males, respectively [16]. The development of liver damages or a fatty liver in both women and men was observed when cholines were absence in diets while the adverse effect was alleviated by supplying sufficient amounts of dietary cholines [17-22]. Also, it was found that bone abnormalities, hemorrhage, renal dysfunction, and growth retardation were developed by fed animals with a choline-deficient diet [23-25]. Therefore, the devoid of ingesting adequate amounts of cholines should risk our health.

A research paper found in the literature reported the results of measuring choline content in 145 commons foods [26]. The authors indicated that among the foods analyzed, the highest levels (mg/100 g) of cholines were as the following: 103 in porks, 116 in dried soybeans, 125 in bacons, 152 in wheat germ, 251 in eggs, 290 in chicken livers, and 418 in beef livers. These results are the sum of sphingomyelins, phosphatidylcholines, glycerophosphocholines, phosphocholines and free cholines in the foods.

Unfortunately, cholines are the deriving sources of trimethylamines that are the deriving sources of trimethylamine N-oxides. Therefore, any food that contains cholines should be regarded as the sources of trimethylamine N-oxides. The most common food components that contain cholines may be phospholipids and carnitines.

L-carnitines are involved in transporting fatty acids into mitochondria in humans or other animals [27]. Unlike the choline, the L-carnitine is not regarded as an essential nutrient. All carnitines required by the body can be endogenously synthesized by utilizing lysines from diets [28-30] though omnivores mainly take up the required L-carnitines from their daily foods. Therefore, the ingestion of carnitines may not be nutritionally needed. L-carnitines mainly exist in such foods as red meats. The high levels of carnitines may also be present in some dietary supplements, and some energy drinks.

It was reported that the level of trimethylamine N-oxides in the blood elevated after the ingestion of foods with the presence of lecithins [5] or carnitines [6] and the gut bacteria that were associated with the conversion of cholines to trimethylamine N-oxides. The control of the carnitine ingestion should not be difficult since it is not an essential nutrient. Since the choline is considered as an essential nutrient, how to find an appropriate way of supplying it is a very challenging task. The ingestion of vegetarian or vegan foods might be a good approach, which seems to be in favor of the gut flora system against the metabolism of carnitines. The control of the gut flora that metabolizes cholin-containing food components to trimethylamines by a clinical intervention might be another feasible way of solving the problem.

In addition to choline-containing food components, trimethylamine N-oxides are present in some aqueous food resources. The trimethylamine N-oxide as an osmolyte is considerably present in saltwater animals, for example, crustaceans, molluscs, rays, and sharks. Although shallow marine animals (except for ureosmotic fishes for example sharks) may contain negligible or at < 100 mmol/kg by wet mass of the trimethylamine N-oxides, it may be upto 300 mmol/kg in deep-sea teleost fishes, skates, certain crustaceans as well as other osmoconforming animals, rising with the depth of the sea [1]. Can trimethylamine N-oxides in these fishes be directly absorbed by the human body? It may also be worth carrying out experiment to illustrate how theyaffect human health.

References

[1] Yancey, P., (2005). Organic osmolytes as compatible, metabolic, and counteracting cytoprotectants in high osmolarity and other stresses. *J. Exp. Biol.* 208(15), 2819–2830.

[2] Elssner, T., Preusser, A., Wagner, U., Kleber, H.P., (1999). Metabolism of L(−)-carnitine by Enterobacteriaceae under aerobic conditions. *FEMS Microbiol. Lett.* 174, 295–301.

[3] Moller, B., Hippe, H., Gottschalk, G., (1986). Degradation of various amine compounds by mesophilic clostridia. *Arch. Microbiol.* 145, 85–90.

[4] Treacy, E.P., Ackerman, B.R., Chow, L.M.L., Youil, R., Bibeau, C., Lin, J., Bruce, A.G., Knight, M., Danks, D.M., Cashman, J.R., Forest, S.M., (1998). Mutations of the flavin-containing monooxygenase gene (FMO3) cause trimethylaminuria, a defect in detoxication. *Hum. Mol. Genet.* 7, 839-845.

[5] Tang, W.H.W., Wang, Z., Levison, B.S., Koeth, R., Britt, E.B., Fu, X.M., Wu, Y.P., Hazen, S.L., (2013). Intestinal microbial metabolism of phosphatidylcholine and cardiovascular risk. *N. Engl. J. Med.* 368(17), 1575-1584.

[6] Wang, Z., Klipfell, E., Bennett, B.J., Koeth, R., Levison, B.S., DuGar, B., Feldstein, A.E., Britt, E.B., Fu, X.M., Chung, Y.M., Wu, Y.P., Schauer, P., Smith, J.D., Allayee, H., Tang, W.H.W., DiDonato, J.A., Lusis, A.J., Hazen, S.L., (2011). Gut flora metabolism of phosphatidylcholine promotes cardiovascular disease. *Nature* 472(7341), 57-63.

[7] Koeth, R.B., Wang, W., Levison, B.S., Buffa, J.A., Org, E., Sheehy, B.T., Britt, E.B., Fu, X.M., Wu, Y.P., Li, L., Smith, J.D., DiDonato, J.A., Chen, J., Li, H.Z., Wu, G.D., Lewis, J.D., Warrier, M., Brown, J.M., Krauss, R.M., Tang, W.H.W., Bushman, F.D., Lusis, A.J., Hazen, S.L., (2013). Intestinal microbiota metabolism of L-carnitine, a nutrient in red meat, promotes atherosclerosis. *Nat. Med.* 19(5), 576-585.

[8] Ufnal, M., Jazwiec, R., Dadlez, M., Drapala, A., Sikora, M., Skrzypecki, J., (2014). Trimethylamine-N-Oxide: A Carnitine-Derived Metabolite That Prolongs the Hypertensive Effect of Angiotensin II in Rats. *Can. J. Cardiol.* 30(12), 1700–1705.

[9] Suzuki, H., Kurihara, Y., Takeya, M., Kamada, N., Kataoka, M., Jishage, K., Ueda, O., Sakaguchi, H., Higashi, T., Suzuki., T., Takashima, Y., Kawabe, Y., Cynshi, O., Wada, Y., Honda, M., Kurihara, H., Aburatani, H., Doi, T., Matsumoto, A., Azuma, S., Noda, T., Toyoda, Y., Itakura, H., Yazaki, Y., Horiuchi, S., Takahashi, K., Kruijt, J.K., van Berkel, T.J.C., Steinbrecher, U.P., Ishibashi, S., Maeda, N., Gordon, S., Kodama, T., (1997). A role for macrophage scavenger receptors in atherosclerosis and susceptibility toinfection. *Nature* 386, 292–296.

[10] Febbraio, M., Podrez, E.A., Smith, J.D., Hajjar, D.P., Hazen, S.L., Hoff, H.F., Sharma, K., Silverstein, R.L., (2000). Targeted disruption of the class B scavenger receptor CD36 protects against atherosclerotic lesion development in mice. *J. Clin. Invest.* 105, 1049–1056.

[11] Zeisel, S.H., da Costa, K.A., (2009). Choline: an essential nutrient for public health. *Nutr. Rev.* 67(11), 615–23.

[12] Zeisel, S.H., (2004). Nutritional importance of choline for brain development. *J. Am. Coll. Nutr.* 23(6), 621S–626S.

[13] Ueland, P.M., (2011). Choline and betaine in health and disease. *J. Inherit. Metab. Dis.* 34(1), 3–15.

[14] Li, Z., Vance, D.E., (2008). Phosphatidylcholine and choline homeostasis. *J. Lipid Res.* 49(6), 1187–1194.

[15] Dumas, M.E., Barton, R.H., Toye, A., Cloarec, O., Blancher, C., Rothwell, A., Fearnside, J., Tatoud, R., Blanc, V., Lindon, J.C., Mitchell, S.C., Holmes, E., McCarthy, M.I., Scott, J., Gauguier, D., Nicholson, J.K., (2006). Metabolic profiling reveals a contribution of gut microbiota to fatty liver phenotype in insulin-resistant mice. *Proc. Natl. Acad. Sci. USA.* 103(33), 12511–12516.

[16] U.S. Department of Agriculture and U.S. Department of Health and Human Services, Dietary Guidelines for Americans, 2010, 7th Edition, Washington, DC: U.S. Government Printing Ofice; December 2010.

[17] Sheard, N.F., Tayek, J.A., Bistrian, B.R., Blackburn, G.L., Zeisel, S.H., (1986). Plasma choline concentration in humans fed parenterally. *Am. J. Clin. Nutr.* 43, 219–224.

[18] Shapira, G., Chawla, R.K., Berry, C.J., Williams, P.J., Roy, R.G.B., Rudman, D., (1986). Cysteine, tyrosine, choline and carnitine supplementation of patients on total parenteral nutrition. *Nutr. Int.* 2, 334–339.

[19] Chawla, R.K., Wolf, D.C., Kutner, M.H., Bonkovsky, H.L., (1989). Choline may be an essential nutrient in malnourished patients with cirrhosis. *Gastroenterol.* 97, 1514–1520.

[20] Buchman, A.L., Moukarzel, A., Jenden, D.J., Roch, M., Rice, K., Ament, M.E., (1993). Low plasma free choline is prevalent in patients receiving long term parenteral nutrition and is associated with hepatic aminotransferase abnor-malities. *Clin. Nutr.* 12, 33–37.

[21] Buchman, A., Dubin, M., Moukarzel, A., Jenden, D., Roch, M., Rice, K., Gornbein, J., Ament, M., (1995). Choline deficiency: a cause of hepatic steatosis during parenteral nutrition that can be reversed with intravenous choline supplementation. *Hepatol.* 22, 1399–1403.

[22] Buchman, A.L., Dubin, M., Jenden, D., Moukarzel, A., Roch, M.H., Rice, K., Gornbein, J., Ament, M.E., Eckhert, C.D., (1992). Lecithin increases plasma free choline and decreases hepatic steatosis in long-term total parenteral nutrition patients. *Gastroenterol.* 102, 1363–1370.

[23] Fairbanks, B.W., Krider, J.L., (1945). Significance of B vitamins in swine nutrition. *N. Am. Vet.* 26, 18–23.

[24] Handler, P., Bernheim, F., (1949). Choline deficiency in the hamster. *Proc. Soc. Exp. Med.* 72, 569.

[25] Newberne, P.M., Rogers, A.E., (1986). Labile methyl groups and the promotion of cancer. *Annu. Rev. Nutr.* 6, 407–432.

[26] Zeisel, S.H., Mar, M.H., Howe, J.C., Holden, J.M., (2003). Concentrations of Choline-Containing Compounds and Betaine in Common Foods. *J. Nutr.* 133, 1302–1307.

[27] Marcovina, S.M., Sirtori, C., Peracino, A., Gheorghiade, M., Borum, P., Remuzzi, G., Ardehali, H., (2013). Translating the basic knowledge of mitochondrial functions to metabolic therapy: role of L-carnitine. *Transl. Res.* 161(2), 73–84.

[28] Bain, M.A., Faull, R., Milne, R.W., Evans, A.M., (2006). Oral L-carnitine: metabolite formation and hemodialysis. *Curr. Drug Metab.* 7(7), 811–816.
[29] Rebouche, C.J., Seim, H., (1998). Carnitine metabolism and its regulation in microorganisms and mammals. *Annu. Rev. Nutr.* 18, 39–61.
[30] Zhang, A.Q., Mitchell, S.C., Smith, R.L., (1999). Dietary precursors of trimethylamine in man: a pilot study. *Food Chem. Toxicol.* 37(5), 515–520.

Chapter 10

Contaminants from Environment

Contaminants in food resources may be defined as those substances that are not produced endogenously, but they are absorbed from the growing environment. The ashes (or minerals, including nutritional and toxic metals) in the food resources are normally accumulated by absorbing from the growing environment.

A proper environment is essential for producing primary food resources. It naturally consists of soil, water, and atmosphere. All these components of the environment can be the source of contaminants.

Food resources can be heavily contaminated by toxic substances if the soil and irrigating water are rich in these undesirables. And also, the food resources that are cultured near to a traffic way can be heavily contaminated by automobile exhaust. For example, it was found that the major vegetables included in diets in Jessore, Bangladesh have the risk high levels of heavy metals [1]. And also, it was reported that soils in the Sundarbans, Bangladesh contain high levels of heavy metals [2]. When food resources are produced in these soils, they can be heavily contaminated by the heavy metals and this might cause a serious health risk if the food resources or animals fed with them are eaten by humans. Furthermore, food resources produced by using an industrial sludge as a soil conditioner or fertilizer could contain high levels of heavy metals [3]. Another report supported this conclusion, which stated that heavy metals can be present in most food products if their growing soil or irrigation water or the aquacultural area contains these metals [4].

Arsenic, lead, mercury, and cadmium are the heavy metals commonly found in food resources and drinking water [5]. How is the significance of these metals in the food resources in term of affecting human health? This question might be interested by any person. Here in this chapter, the effects of these four heavy metals on the cardiovascular system are concentrated on.

Arsenic

As (III), e.g. As_2O_3, and As (V), e.g. As_2O_5, are the main states of arsenic though it can also exist in other valence states. As_2O_3, and As_2O_5 are soluble in water to become weak acidic solutions. As (III) and As (V) are inter-convertible via redox reaction. Both inorganic forms just mentioned above of the arsenic are toxic. As (III) is more toxic than As (V). The arsenic can also exist in an organic form, which is less toxic than the inorganic form.

The inorganic arsenic compounds (including As (III) as well as As(V)) are able to be taken up by the human body and accumulate in body fluids and tissues [6]. The normal level of these compounds can be converted into a cacodylic acid or dimethylarsinic acid (accounting for $\geq$ 90% of the metabolites) via the non-enzymatic or enzymatic methylation in the liver of mammals and excreted with the urine [7].

However, the adverse health effect caused by the chronic toxicity of arsenics appears to be a publicly important issue in Japan, Hungary, Argentina, Chile, Bangladesh, India, or China [8]. Especially, it was reported that dietary arsenics can increase CVD risks [9] though arsenics may also cause other health problems. Exposures to inorganic arsenics because of occupation or environment were found to be positively associated with the elevated mortality of CVDs [10,11]. Clinical investigations also indicated that inorganic arsenics were dose-dependently associated with strokes, coronary heart diseases, atherosclerosis, hypertension, and diabetes mellitus [12,13]. Epidemiologic investigations also indicated a correlation between chronic exposures (low to moderate doses) to arsenics by drinking water and CVDs in the US [14,15]. Chronic exposures to arsenics by drinking water cumulatively resulted in greater incidence of ischemic heart diseases in individuals, as compared with control individuals after the adjustment of multivariate factors [12]. This conclusion is supported by the fact that the termination of consuming well water rich in arsenics reduced the mortality of ischemic heart diseases in southwestern Taiwan [16]. Furthermore, chronic exposures to arsenics resulted in the greater morbidity of hypertension among residents living in endemic areas, comparing to those living in nonendemic areas in Bangladesh [17]. Another study found the association of exposures to inorganic arsenics by drinking water with an elevated risk of inducing type 2 diabetes mellitus, which was not caused by the cumulative effect of exposures to arsenics [18]. Drinking water rich in arsenics resulted in an increase in the mortality of acute myocardial infarctions in Chile while the remediation of an arsenic exposure alleviated the adverse effect [19].

The accumulation of arsenics in the blood vessel wall usually coexists with the formation of atherosclerotic lesions and an increased macrophage accumulation and fibrosis [9]. Drinking water rich in sodium arsenite caused arsenics accumulating in the wall of vessels and elevated the formation of atherosclerotic lesions in the aorta of female mice with ApoE-knockout without the elevation of cholesterols in plasma. The mice with exposures to arsenics developed the atherosclerotic lesions and had elevated fibrosis and the accumulation of macrophages, comparing with the control drinking water low in arsenics [20]. The mechanism of increasing atherosclerosis risks by exposures to arsenics might involve the promotion of oxidative stresses, vascular inflammation, some reactive oxidants and apoptosis.

For the mechanism of developing atherosclerosis involving oxidative stresses, it was found that the reactive oxygen species were increased by exposures to arsenics [21]. *In vitro* investigations indicated that hydrogen peroxides (H_2O_2), superoxides, and oxidants were produced by exposures to arsenics [22]. Another study also found that the level of arsenics in blood was positively associated with the plasma level of hydrogen peroxides, reactive oxidants (superoxide (O_2^-), and the reduced antioxidative capacity [23]. These findings may support the opinion on the association of oxidative stresses induced by exposures to arsenics with the increased risk of CVDs, such as atherosclerosis. The oxidation of lipids may result from the oxidative stresses. Lipids that were oxidized were found in every stage of atherogenesis, which could produce isoprostanes, peroxides, and other bioactive molecules with aldehydes (4-hydroxy-trans-2-nonenal and malondialdehyde) being the main end products [24]. An investigation into animals found that there was an elevation of plasma concentrations of free lipid aldehydes and their protein adducts accumulated in atherosclerotic lesions [25]. It should be believable that the formation of atherosclerotic lesions was exacerbated by exposures to arsenics which resulted in the excessive level of highly reactive lipid aldehydes and the subsequent elevation of lipid uptake by scavenger receptors, cytokine production, and monocyte adhesion, or reduced detoxification [26].

The inflammation can also be caused by oxidative stresses, which could then increase the risk of atherosclerosis. For the mechanism of developing atherosclerosis associated with inflammation, it was found that the *in vitro* administration of sodium arsenite resulted in the expression of proinflammatory cytokines such as IL-6 and monocyte MCP-1, and chemokines in vascular lesions [27]. Another study also found that exposures to arsenics elevated the expression of circulating lymphocyte MCP-1 mRNA and the concentration of MCP-1 in plasma in humans [28]. Furthermore, it was reported that the elevation of exposures to arsenics elevated several growth factors and cytokines that were associated with inflammation in individuals [28]. It was also found that there was a positive correlation between the concentrations of arsenics in serum and the concentrations of endothelial dysfunction (also possibly caused by inflammation) or systemic inflammation markers (for example, SVCAM-1 and SICAM-1) in plasma in subjects living in Bangladesh [29,30]. It was reported that CVDs were well predicted by the markers of endothelial dysfunction as well as systemic inflammation [31]. This is supported by another report that indicated the involvement of inflammation in the pathophysiology of atherosclerosis [32]. Moreover, the development of carotid atherosclerosis was observed in individuals with the genotypes of ApoE and MCP1 who drank the water rich in arsenics [33].

The association of exposures to arsenics with diabetes may involve an adverse effect on the respiration in cells by inhibiting several saccharides enzymes (i.e., the pathways of glycolysis or gluconeogenesis) and the uncoupled oxidative phosphorylation [35]. However, other mechanisms, such as apoptosis, inflammation, oxidative stresses, or nonspecific mechanisms may also be involved in the association of exposures to arsenics with type 2 diabetes [32]. The acute toxicity of exposures to arsenics may adversely affect the expression of factors, which are associated with the pathways of insulin (for example, upstream factor 1 of insulin in the cells of pancreas or peroxisome proliferator-activated receptor γ in preadipocytes), for gene transcription and therefore increases the risk of diabetes [9].

It seems that no report on the association of ingesting organic arsenics with the development of CVDs can be found in the literature. And also, it appears to be difficult of finding a report that denies their association with CVDs in the literature. Therefore, it would be worth carrying out investigations into the possibility of their association with CVDs.

Lead

Pb(II) and Pb(IV) are the main states of lead naturally existing while Pb(II) is more common than Pb(IV). Pb(IV) may not be involved in dietary toxicity since it can only exist in strong acidic solution [36]. Leads can be dissolved in organic acid solutions with the existence of oxygen and lead bicarbonate is also quite soluble in water.

Exposures to leads in humans may result from water, foods and atmosphere. The lead-contamination of foods mainly originates from food manufacturing, growing soil, agriculture practices and pollution from the industry. Solder of cans for holding foods or beverages as well as glazed ceramics for storing or preparing foods and beverages could also be significant sources of lead contamination. The lead-contaminating sources of water should be much more than those of foods.

The levels $\geq$10 μg/dL of blood leads were considered as being toxic in young children by the CDC statement whereas a new guideline for treating the concentrations $\geq$15 μg/dL of blood leads was also recommended [37]. Nevertheless, adequate evidences seem to show that the poisoning index just mentioned above may be too high for applying to adults [38].

Chronic exposures to leads are associated with atherosclerosis, peripheral arterial diseases, strokes, coronary heart diseases, hypertension [39], and the mortality or morbidity of CVDs [40]. These CVDs have the potential of threatening a life. For example, it was reported that studying animals developed atherosclerosis because of lead toxicity [41]. Furthermore, the elevated mortality of CVDs and atherosclerosis in men were found to be associated with chronic exposures to leads [42]. Epidemiological investigations found that peripheral artery diseases, hypertension and other illness outcomes were positively linked to exposures to the low levels of leads in a graded manner [43-45].

The elevation of oxidative stresses may be associated with the mechanism of leads causing CVDs. For example, epidemiological investigations into individuals with high lead exposures because of their occupation indicated the involvement of markers of oxidative stresses in lead toxicity [46]. A cycle of inflammation and oxidative stresses in the target tissues might be triggered by the production of reactive oxygen species promoted by exposures to leads [47]. Redox-inactive metals were reported to induce oxidative stresses that might be indirectly associated with the depletion, which might be linked to CVDs, of major sulfhydryl reserves in cells [48]. The mechanism of inducing hypertension by exposures to leads may also be associated with increased oxidative stresses [49]. Reactive oxygen species (O_2^-) are able to inactivate NO, which may result in an increase in blood pressure. This is supported by the fact that NO availability in rats elevated by the supplementation of ascorbic acids and vitamin Es (an antioxidant therapy) in control rats and no impact on nitrotyrosines (the marker of NO oxidation) in tissues or blood pressure because of exposures to leads were observed [50]. Decreases in the bioavailability of NO by exposures to leads might impair the tone of vasomotor which could be a risk factor for atherosclerosis and hypertension. NO may physiologically have multiple effects on vascular walls, such as endothelium-mediating vasodilatation, inhibiting the activation of platelets, the proliferation and migration of smooth muscle cells, and the inactivation of the NF-κB that suppresses the proinflammatory mediators [51]. For example, the NFκB was also found to be activated by exposures to leads, which might be partially involved in inducing hypertension [52]. The results of oxidative stresses resulted from exposures to leads have been mostly indicated by *in vitro* studies [53] or investigations into animals [54]. It was also assumed that exposures to leads were associated with the induction of vasoconstriction that was mediated by an alpha adrenoceptor, which could result in hypertension [55]. Blood pressure may also be increased by elevating the production of angiotensin and renin because of nephrotoxicity of leads [56]. The impaired function of renals caused by exposures to leads may be the major reason for hypertension since it had been found that the concentrations < 5μg/dL of leads in blood were inversely associated with the measured rate of glomerular filtration in general population [38].

There are other mechanisms that may be potentially involved in the association of lead toxicity with CVDs. For example, chronic exposures to leads were found to have an effect on the mechanical and electrical activity of the heart and to change the function of vascular smooth muscles while the cardiac function was affected by acute exposures to leads [57]. It was also suggested that the multiple sites of the cardiovascular system are targeted by leads [58]. Other studies indicated that the systemic metabolism of lipids might be affected by chronic exposures to leads [41]. The inflammation caused by exposures to leads may also be involved in the mechanism of inducing the development of CVDs to some degrees [32]. This might be supported by the fact that exposures to leads elevated the expression or production of markers of inflammation in humans [59]. In addition to the association of inflammation and oxidative stresses [60], impaired NO homeostasis [61], and others that have been discussed above, the promotion of transformation and proliferation of vascular smooth muscle cells may also be involved in the mechanism of lead toxicity. The alteration of calcium metabolism caused by exposures to leads was also suggested to be involved in the mechanism of changing vascular resistance and inducing hypertension [62]. The reason for this may be that leads are in competition with calciums for the pumps and channels of transporting ions across the cell membranes and between the mitochondria, endoplasmic reticulum, and cytoplasm, and this therefore results in the variation of cytosolic calcium ions involving in the contraction of vascular smooth muscles and the adjustment of vascular tone [63]. Moreover, the control of contraction of vascular smooth muscles, which is mediated by calciums, might be adversely affected by leads through replacing calciums in signaling pathways involving in the interaction of calmodulin and calcium, and potassium channels that are dependent on calciums [64]. Calcium ions were reported to be freely released by the mitochondria because of the imbalance between the counteraction by the antioxidative defenses in cells and the production of free radicals caused by oxidative stresses [65]. The adverse effect of leads on the contraction of smooth muscles and the intercellular messengers (protein kinase C) may elevate the pressor responsiveness to catecholamines, which might also be involved in the mechanism of cardiovascular toxicity of exposures to leads [66].

Clinical investigations appear to give controversial results in term of correlation between the concentrations of leads in the blood and the incidence of CVDs [44,67,68]. The variation of findings might result from the variations of investigation cohorts with factors of toxicokinetics/exposures (e.g., amount, duration), characteristics of the environment (e.g., setting of assessment, supports of development, coexistence of morbidity or exposures), characteristics (having an effect on lead metabolism) of genes, and background of races or the health state of subjects [69,70].

Mercury

Three forms of the mercury can be found in nature, which include inorganic mercury compounds, organic mercury compounds, and metallic or elemental mercury. Hg (I) and Hg(II) are the main oxidation states though higher oxidation states may also exist [71]. Hg(II) is more common than Hg(I) in nature.

The mercury in forms that are fat- or water-soluble (for example methylmercury or mercuric chloride) should be the main source of dietary exposures that may result in poisoning. The mercury can be acutely and chronically toxic. Organic mercury compounds are the most poisonous forms, e.g. methylmercury. The safe daily ingestion of the methylmercury was recommended to be < 0.1μg/kg body weight [72].

Naturally, the mercury tends to accumulate in shellfishes and fishes, which is mainly in the form of the methylmercury. This form of the mercury is highly poisonous. Fishes on the higher trophic level of a food chain usually contain greater levels of the mercury, as compared to those on the lower trophic level. The mecury content in sharks, tilefishes, albacore tunas, bluefin tunas, king mackerels, and swordfishes is higher than in others. The fat soluble methylmercury and other forms of the mercury mainly deposit in the viscera though they are also present in all muscle tissues [73]. The accumulation of the methylmercury is more efficient than its depuration so that its content in fishes rises as the time goes on.

The cardiovascular toxicity of the mercury is likely to be associated with oxidative damages, hypertension, and other CVDs (such as CHDs or myocardial infarctions). This conclusion is based on many established scientific evidences. For example, it was reported that the mercury plays a role in the development of strokes, hypertension, and other cardiovascular diseases in humans [74]. It was confirmed that an elevated development of atherosclerosis and risk of CVDs were found to be linked to the high concentration of the mercury in hairs [75]. Both *in vitro* and *in vivo* studies showed the development of atherosclerosis induced by an exposure to the mercury [76,77]. It was also reported that the beneficial impacts of ingesting fishes on the health of the cardiovascular system might be eliminated by the high concentration of the mercury in them [78]. The mercury was found to be potentially associated with the development of CVDs [79], which was supported by the results of several follow-up investigations [80,81]. These findings are further supported by the association of an exposure to the mercury vapor via amalgam in dentists with the elevated risk of CVDs [82]. A prospective investigation carried out in Sweden found a controversial result, i.e. the adverse association of the blood mercury and polyunsaturated fatty acids with myocardial infarctions [83]. However, the authors also claimed that the concentrations of the mercury in the blood was very low and the mercury was unlikely to have a protective effect on the cardiovascular system. Furthermore, the authors did not tell how many years the investigations were undertaken and the sampling time of the blood for the determination of mercury content.

The limitation of data that are available might be the reason for the uncertainties in relation to the association of the mercury with diabetes mellitus and hypertension [84,85]. A case report and literature review suggested the association of the mercury intoxication with arterial hypertension [86]. Review papers published in 2011 and 2012 stated that the association of hypertension in humans with the mercury poisoning is undoubted [74,87]. However, a research paper published in 2012 concluded that the exposure to the methylmercury did not clinically increase the risk of hypertension in women or men, covering geometric average toenail levels of 740 μg/kg in the highest quintile and 80 μg/kg in the lowest quintile [88].

The mechanism of the association of the exposure to the mercury with CVDs may be involved in the induction of oxidative stresses [89], apoptosis and the alteration of function of mitochondria [90], and the depletion of sulfhydryl groups [91]. Both *in vitro* and *in vivo* studies showed the induction of oxidative impairment of tissues (e.g. myocardia) by the exposure to the mercury. The exposure to the mercury may elevate the production of reactive oxygen species or lower the ability of antioxidative defenses. For example, it was found that both nonenzymatic and enzymatic antioxidants were able to alleviate the toxicity of the methylmercury [92]. It should be noted that there is currently a lack of information of mercury-induced oxidative damages to the cardiovascular system in relation to humans. Furthermore, the mercury is capable of binding to compounds that contain thiol groups, for example, glutathione [93] and therefore decreasing the ability of antioxidative defenses. It seems that the mercury is primarily carried and removed from the body in the form of glutathione-mercury complexes and this would further reduce the ability of antioxidative defenses in cells. *In vitro* investigations also suggested that the thiol groups in the platelet membranes bound by the mercury were able to induce the alteration of platelet aggregation [94]. In addition, the mercury is also able to form an insoluble complex with selenium. The interaction between the mercury and the selenium or thiol-containing compounds would be able to increase the peroxidation of lipids and the stress of free radicals and decrease the capacity of antioxidative defenses in the human body [79]. Another possible mechanism may involve that the mercury was found to be capable of altering the integrity of structure of the inner membranes in mitochondria and therefore causing the loss of selectivity of normal cations [77]. More suggested possible mechanisms of mercury toxicity may be associated with the inhibition of activating NF-κB which increases the peroxidation of lipids and consecutively elevates the risk of developing atherosclerosis. The sulfhydryl groups of NF-κB may be bound by the mercury, and this would cause the impaired activation of NF-κB which subsequently reduces its impacts on the expression of genes [95]. The inhibition of pathway of NF-κB was found to reduce the production of NO by *in vitro* investigations via the inactivation of expression of inducible NO synthase genes [96]. The NO production is catalyzed by NO synthases, which is vital for maintaining the immune system and vascular regulation [97].

Cadmium

The cadmium is a metal that is bluish-white divalent, ductile, malleable, and soft, and analogous to a zinc in many aspects except for forming complex compounds [98]. Cd(II) is the main oxidation state though Cd(I) also exists. It can form many complex compounds with such organic compounds as vitamins, amino acids, nucleobases, and proteins [99].

Dietary exposures to cadmiums mainly include the ingestion of foods that are contaminated (such as crustaceans, offals, molluscs, algal products, organ meats, grains, leafy vegetables, tubers, starchy roots) as well as drinking water. It has been recommended by EFSA that the tolerable weekly intake of cadmiums for humans is 2.5 μg/kg body weight [100]. The Joint FAO/WHO Expert Committee on Food Additives has recommended a provisional tolerable monthly intake level for cadmiums of 25 μg/kg body weight [101]. The guideline value of cadmiums in water was recommended to be < 0.3 μg/L [102].

Chronic exposures to cadmiums were reported to be linked to diabetes and hypertension [103,104]. It was found that the adverse alterations of the vessel walls might be initiated by the low-dose of cadmiums (< their known toxic levels) [105]. The level of cadmiums in the blood was found to be potentially associated with an increased blood pressure though correlation between hypertension and urinary cadmiums was not found [106]. Epidemiological investigations indicated that patients with diabetes were highly susceptible to the development of cadmium-induced dysfunction of renals [107]. Another investigation showed that the high concentrations of cadmiums in urine were significantly associated with the high concentrations of fasting glucoses in the blood being dependent of doses, and that the diabetic patients were more susceptible to the adverse impacts resulted from exposures to cadmiums [108].

Investigations into animals and *in vitro* trials also observed the adverse effects of cadmiums on the cardiovascular system [109,110]. Furthermore, male patients with CVDs from the areas where there was a potential increased exposures to cadmiums were found to have elevated mortality, which might imply that the cadmium should be at least a part of factors for morbidity though this result could not tell whether it was a cause or not [111]. It was also found that the thickening (measured by intimamedia thickness ratio) of early atherosclerotic vessel walls [112] and myocardial infarctions [113] were linked to the level of cadmiums in the blood independent of other factors. The adverse effects of cadmiums on the cardiovascular system were suggestive of including the induction of disadvantageous alterations of cardiac function or metabolism and the promotion of atherosclerosis [114].

There are also minor reports that give some controversial results in relation to the relationship between cadmiums and the risk of CVDs. For example, it was reported that the level of cadmiums in the blood was not associated with the estimated function of arteria [115]. The different results reported may be caused by the variations of strengths in different investigations. For example some investigations had a strong design of prospective studies [116], and the measures of blood pressure being a continuous variable without misclassifying bias of outcomes [117], some others had the limitation of small size of samples, un-adjusting potential confounders, un-standardizing the measures of blood pressure [106]. The improper selection of samples and the error of measures of exposures might be the additional weakness in these studies [118].

The mechanism of the association of exposures to cadmiums with CVDs might be involved in the following aspects: inhibiting the production of vasodilator compounds for example NO, partially activating the channels of calciums, directly vasoconstricting [119], promoting the oxidative stresses [110], depleting the glutathione [120], altering sulfhydryl homeostasis [120], indirectly elevating oxidative stresses and the peroxidation of lipids [121], moving into the vessel wall [122], being absorbed by the immune system [122], depositing on the vascular wall, disrupting the endothelial integrity, stimulating the proliferation of smooth muscle cells, and causing the death of cells. Another study supported the promotion of oxidative stresses in endothelial cells by exposures to cadmiums [123], and depositing on the vascular wall [124]. In addition to cadmiums being directly taken up by endocytosis and thus moving to cells in the wall of vessels, cells in the immune system may also take up cadmiums, infiltrating and entering the wall of vessels, such as, by cadmium-laden monocytes [122]. This process is likely to produce foam cells and causes the death of necrotic foam cells, which might initiate and promote the development of atherosclerosis. Furthermore, the disruption of the endothelial integrity might also be induced by cadmiums and the subsequent uptake of cadmiums could result in the death of endothelial cells. This process could usually cause gaps between endothelial cells, facilitating the diffusion of cadmiums from the stream of blood into the medial layer [125]. It seems that cadmiums could be sufficiently transported across the endothelium of cells of vascular walls and the high levels of cadmiums could mainly remain in smooth muscle cells [124]. The low level of cadmiums could also affect Ca^{2+} flux and ion homeostasis, be cytotoxic, and stimulate the proliferation of smooth muscle cells [126], which therefore facilitate lipids subsequently accumulating in the wall of vessels and modify lipid profiles to be more atherogenic [32]. It was also reported that cadmiums are capable of fundamentally promoting atherosclerosis by inducing the death of endothelial cells [125].

The metallothionein-cadmium complex is the main transporting form of cadmiums in the blood. This process can alleviate oxidative stresses or other toxicities caused by cadmiums. However, this might not be able to deal the over-loading of cadmiums in the blood. Several transporters and ion channels were found to carry cadmiums across plasma membranes, such as plasma membrane-associated duodenal metal transporter-1 [127] and calcium-channels [128]. Whether these mechanisms are associated with the development of CVDs or not needs further study to illustrate.

References

[1] Alam, M.G.M., Snow, E.T., Tanaka, A., (2003). Arsenic and heavy metal contamination of vegetables grown in Samta Village, Bangladesh. *Sci. Total Environ.* 308 (1-3), 83-96.

[2] Awal, M.A., Hale, W.H.G., Stern, B., (2009). Trace element concentrations in mangrove sediments in the Sundarbans, Bangladesh. *Mar. Poll. Bull.* 58(12), 1944-1948.

[3] Islam, M.M., Halim, M.A., Safiullah, S., Hoque, S.A.M.W., Islam, M.S., (2009). Heavy metal content in textile sludge in Gazipur, Bangladesh. *Res. J. Environ. Sci.* 3 (3), 311-315.

[4] De Vries, W., Römkens, P.F.A.M., Schütze, G., (2007). Critical soil concentrations of cadmium, lead, and mercury in view of health effects on humans and animals. *Rev. Environ. Contam. Toxicol.* 191, 91-130.

[5] Järup, L., (2003). Hazards of heavy metal contamination. *Br. Med. Bull.* 68(1), 167-182.

[6] Ueki, K., Kondo, T., Tseng, Y.H., Kahn, C.R., (2004). Central role of suppressors of cytokine signaling proteins in hepatic steatosis, insulin resistance, and the metabolic syndrome in the mouse. *Proceed. Nat. Acad. Sci. USA* 101(28), 10422–7.

[7] Vigo, J.B., Ellzey, J.T., (2006). Effects of Arsenic Toxicity at the Cellular Level: A Review. *Texas J. Microsc.* 37(2), 45–49.

[8] Smith, A.H., Smith, M.M.H., (2004). Arsenic drinking water regulations in developing countries with extensive exposure. *Toxicol.* 198, 39–44.

[9] Alissa, E.M, Ferns, G.A., (2011). Heavy metal poisoning and cardiovascular disease. *J. Toxicol.* 2011, 870125. 21pages. doi:10.1155/2011/870125

[10] Tsai, S.M., Wang, T.N., Ko, Y.C., (1999). Mortality for certain diseases in areas with high levels of arsenic in drinking water. *Arch. Environ. Health* 54(3), 186–193.

[11] Axelson, O., Dahlgren, E., Jansson, C.D., Rehnlund, S.O., (1978). Arsenic exposure and mortality: a case referent study from a Swedish copper smelter. *Brit. J. Industr. Med.* 35(1), 8–15.

[12] Tseng, C.H., Chong, C.K., Tseng, C.P., Hsueh, Y.M., Chiou, H.Y., Tseng, C.C., Chen, C.J., (2003). Long-term arsenic exposure and ischemic heart disease in arseniasis-hyperendemic villages inTaiwan. *Toxicol. Lett.* 137(1-2), 15–21.

[13] Chiou, H.Y., Huang, W.I., Su, C.L., Chang, S.F., Hsu, Y.H., Chen, C.J., (1997). Dose-response relationship between prevalence of cerebrovascular disease and ingested inorganic arsenic. *Stroke* 28(9), 1717–1723.

[14] Meliker, J.R., Wahl, R.L., Cameron, L.L., Nriagu, J.O., (2007). Arsenic in drinking water and cerebrovascular disease, diabetes mellitus, and kidney disease in Michigan: a standardized mortality ratio analysis. *Environ. Health* 6, article 4.

[15] Zierold, K.M., Knobeloch, L., Anderson, H., (2004). Prevalence of chronic diseases in adults exposed to arsenic-contaminated drinking water. *Am. J. Pub. Health* 94(11), 1936–1937.

[16] Chang, C.C., Ho, S.C., Tsai, S.S., Yang, C.Y., (2004). Ischemic heart disease mortality reduction in an arseniasis-endemic area in southwestern Taiwan after a switch in the tap-water supply system. *J. Toxicol. Environ. Health Part A* 67(17), 1353–1361.

[17] Rahman, M., Tondel, M., Ahmad, S.A., Chowdhury, I.A., Faruquee, M.H., Axelson, O., (1999). Hypertension and arsenic exposure in Bangladesh. *Hypertens.* 33(1), 74–78.

[18] Tseng, C.H., Tai, T.Y., Chong, C.K., Tseng, C.P., Lai, M.S., Lin, B.J., Chiou, H.Y., Hsueh, Y.M., Hsu, K.H., Chen, C.J., (2000). Long-term arsenic exposure and incidence of non-insulin-dependent diabetes mellitus: a cohort study in arseniasis-hyperendemic villages in Taiwan. *Environ. Health Persp.* 108(9), 847–851.

[19] Yuan, Y., Marshall, G., Ferreccio, C., Steinmaus, C., Selvin, S., Liaw, J., Bates, M.N., Smith, A.H., (2007). Acute myocardial infarction mortality in comparison with lung and bladder cancer mortality in arsenic-exposed region II of Chile from 1950 to 2000. *Am. J. Epidemiol.* 166(12), 1381–1391.

[20] Simeonova, P.P., Hulderman, T., Harki, D., Luster, M.I., (2003). Arsenic exposure accelerates atherogenesis in apolipoprotein E(-/-) mice. *Environ. Health Persp.* 111(14), 1744–1748.

[21] Barchowsky, A., Klei, L.R., Dudek, E.J., Swartz, H.M., James, P.E., (1999).Stimulation of reactive oxygen, but not reactive nitrogen species, in vascular endothelial cells exposed to low levels of arsenite. *Free Rad. Biol. Med.* 27(11-12), 1405–1412.

[22] Lee, T.C., Ho, I.C., (1995). Modulation of cellular antioxidant defense activities by sodium arsenite in human fibroblasts. *Arch. Toxicol.* 69(7), 498–504.

[23] Wu, M.M., Chiou, H.Y., Wang, T.W., Hsueh, Y.M., Wang, I.H., Chen, C.J., Lee, T.C., (2001). Association of arsenic exposure with increased reactive oxidants and decreased antioxidant capacity in a human population of Northeastern Taiwan. *Environ. Health Persp.* 109(10), 1011–1017.

[24] Esterbauer, H., Schaur, R.J., Zollner, H., (1991). Chemistry and biochemistry of 4-hydroxynonenal, malonaldehyde and related aldehydes. *Free Rad. Biol. Med.* 11(1), 81–128.

[25] Rosenfeld, M.E., Ross, R., (1990). Macrophage and smooth muscle cell proliferation in atherosclerotic lesions of WHHL and comparably hypercholesterolemic fat-fed rabbits. *Arterioscler.* 10(5), 680–687.

[26] Santra, A., Maiti, A., Das, S., Lahiri, S., Charkaborty, S.K., Mazumder, D.N., (2000). Hepatic damage caused by chronic arsenic toxicity in experimental animals. *J. Toxicol. Clin. Toxicol.* 38(4), 395–405.

[27] Lee, P.C., Ho, I.C., Lee, T.C., (2005). Oxidative stress mediates sodium arsenite-induced expression of heme oxygenase-1, monocyte chemoattractant protein-1, and interleukin-6 in vascular smooth muscle cells. *Toxicol. Sci.* 85(1), 541–550.

[28] Wu, M.M., Chiou, H.Y., Ho, I.C., Chen, C.J., Lee, T.C., (2003). Gene expression of inflammatory molecules in circulating lymphocytes from arsenic-exposed human subjects. *Environ. Health Persp.* 111(11), 1429–1438.

[29] Chen, Y., Santella, R.M., Kibriya, M.G., Wang, Q., Kappil, M., Verret, W.J., Graziano, J.H., Ahsan, H., (2007). Association between arsenic exposure from drinking water and plasma levels of soluble cell adhesion molecules. *Environ. Health Persp.* 115(10), 1415–1420.

[30] Wu, F., Jasmine, F., Kibriya, M.G., Liu, M., Wójcik, O., Parvez, F., Rahaman, R., Roy, S., Paul-Brutus, R., Segers, S., Slavkovich, V., Islam, T., Levy, D., Mey, J.L., van Geen, A.,Graziano, J.H., Ahsan, H., Chen, Y., (2012). Association between arsenic exposure from drinking water and plasma levels of cardiovascular markers. *Am. J. Epidemiol.* 175(12), 1252-61.

[31] Ridker, P.M., Hennekens, C.H., Roitman-Johnson, B., Stampfer, M.J., Allen, J., (1998). Plasma concentration of soluble intercellular adhesionmolecule 1 and risks of future myocardial infarction in apparently healthy men. *Lancet.* 351(9096), 88–92.

[32] Ross, R., (1999). Atherosclerosis—an inflammatory disease. *N. Engl. J. Med.* 340, 115–126.

[33] Hsieh, Y.C., Hsieh, F.I., Lien, L.M., Chou, Y.L., Chiou, H.Y., Chen, C.J., (2008). Risk of carotid atherosclerosis associated with genetic polymorphisms of apolipoprotein E and inflammatory genes among arsenic exposed residents in Taiwan. *Toxicol. Appl. Pharmacol.* 227(1), 1–7.

[34] Waalkes, M.P., Fox, D.A., States, J.C., Patierno, S.R., McCabe, M.J., (2000). Metals and disorders of cell accumulation: modulation of apoptosis and cell proliferation. *Toxicol. Sci.* 56(2), 255–261.

[35] Patlolla, A.K., Tchounwou, P.B., (2005). Serum acetyl cholinesterase as a biomarker of arsenic induced neurotoxicity in sprague-dawley rats. *Intern. J. Environ. Res. Pub. Health* 2(1), 80–83.

[36] Polyanskiy, N.G., In: Fillipova, N.A, ed. Аналитическая химия элементов: Свинец [*Analytical Chemistry of the Elements: Lead*] (in Russian). Nauka; 1986.

[37] CDC (Centers for Disease Control and Prevention), Preventing Lead Poisoning in Young Children: A Statement by the Centers for Disease Control. US Departmentof Health and Human Services, Atlanta, Ga, USA; 1991.

[38] Muntner, P., Menke, A., DeSalvo, K.B., Rabito, F.A., Batuman, V., (2005). Continued decline in blood lead levels among adults in the United States: the National Health and Nutrition Examination Surveys. *Arch. Intern. Med.* 165(18), 2155–2161.

[39] Nawrot, T.S., Thijs, L., DenHond, E.M., Roels, H.A., Staessen, J.A., (2002). An epidemiological re-appraisal of the association between blood pressure and blood lead: a meta-analysis. *J. Hum. Hypertens.* 16(2), 123–131.

[40] Schwartz, J., (1995). Lead, blood pressure, and cardiovascular disease in men. *Arch. Environ. Health* 50(1), 31–37.

[41] Revis, N.W., Zinsmeister, A.R., Bull, R., (1981). Atherosclerosis and hypertension induction by lead and cadmium ions: an effect prevented by calcium ion. *Proceed. Nat. Acad. Sci. USA* 78(10), 6494–6498.

[42] Schober, S.E., Mirel, L. B., Graubard, B.I., Brody, D.J., Flegal, K.M., (2006). Blood lead levels and death from all causes, cardiovascular disease, and cancer: results from the NHANES III Mortality Study. *Environ. Health Persp.* 114(10), 1538–1541.

[43] Lee, D.H., Lim, J.S., Song, K., Boo, Y., Jacobs, D.R., (2006). Graded associations of blood lead and urinary cadmium concentrations with oxidative stress related markers in the U.S. population: results from the third National Health and Nutrition Examination Survey. *Environ. Health Persp.* 114(3), 350–354.

[44] Navas-Acien, A., Selvin, E., Sharrett, A.R., Calderon-Aranda, E., Silbergeld, E., Guallar, E., (2004). Lead, cadmium, smoking, and increased risk of peripheral arterial disease. *Circulation* 109(25), 3196–3201.

[45] Nash, D., Magder, L., Lustberg, M., Sherwin, R.W., Rubin, R.J., Kaufmann, R.B., Silbergeld, E.K., (2003). Blood lead, blood pressure, and hypertension in perimenopausal and post-menopausal women. *J. Am. Med. Assoc.* 289(12), 1523–1532.

[46] Kasperczyk, S., Birkner, E., Kasperczyk, A., Kasperczyk, J., (2005). Lipids, lipid peroxidation and 7-ketocholesterol in workers exposed to lead. *Hum. Exper. Toxicol.* 24(6), 287–295.

[47] Gonick, H.C., Ding, Y., Bondy, S.C., Ni, Z., Vaziri, N.D., (1997). Lead-induced hypertension: interplay of nitric oxide and reactive oxygen species. *Hypertens.* 30(6), 1487–1492.

[48] Ercal, N., Gurer-Orhan, H., Aykin-Burns, N., (2001). Toxic metals and oxidative stress part I: mechanisms involved in metal-induced oxidative damage. *Curr. Top. Med. Chem.* 1(6), 529–539.

[49] Vaziri, N.D., Lin, C.Y., Farmand, F., Sindhu, R.K., (2003). Superoxide dismutase, catalase, glutathione peroxidase and NADPH oxidase in lead-induced hypertension. *Kidney Intern.* 63(1), 186–194.

[50] Vaziri, N.D., Liang, K., Ding, Y., (1999). Increased nitric oxide inactivation by reactive oxygen species in lead induced hypertension. *Kidney Intern.* 56(4), 1492– 1498.

[51] Libby, P., (2000). Changing concepts of atherogenesis. *J. Intern. Med.* 247(3), 349–358.

[52] Rodríguez-Iturbe, B., Sindhu, R.K., Quiroz, Y., Vaziri, N.D., (2005). Chronic exposure to low doses of lead results in renal infiltration of immune cells, NF-κB activation, and over-expression of tubulointerstitial angiotensin II. *Antioxid. Redox Sign.* 7(9-10), 1269–1274.

[53] Ding, Y., Gonick, H.C., Vaziri, N.D., (2000). Lead promotes hydroxyl radical generation and lipid peroxidation in cultured aortic endothelial cells. *Am. J. Hypertens.* 13(5), 552–555.

[54] Fowler, B.A., Whittaker, M.H., Lipsky, M., Wang, G., Chen, X.Q., (2004). Oxidative stress induced by lead, cadmium and arsenic mixtures: 30-day, 90-day, and 180-day drinking water studies in rats: an overview. *BioMet.* 17(5), 567–568.

[55] Bertel, O., Buehler, F.R., Ott, J., (1978). Lead-induced hypertension: blunted beta-adrenoceptor-mediated functions. *Brit. Med. J.* 1(6112), 551.

[56] Jhaveri, R.C., Lavorgna, L., Dube, S.K., Glass, L., Khan, F., Evans, H.E., (1979). Relationship of blood pressure to blood lead concentrations in small children. *Pediatrics* 63(4), 674–676.

[57] Kopp, S.J., Barron, J.T., Tow, J.P., (1988). Cardiovascular actions of lead and relationship to hypertension: a review. *Environ. Health Persp.* 78, 91–99.

[58] Prentice, R.C., Kopp, S.J., (1985). Cardiotoxicity of lead at various perfusate calcium concentrations: functional and metabolic responses of the perfused rat heart. *Toxicol. Appl. Pharmacol.* 81(3), 491–501.

[59] Mishra, K.P., Singh, V.K., Rani, R., Yadav, V.S., Chandran, V., Srivastava, S.P., Seth, P.K., (2003). Effect of lead exposure on the immune response of some occupationally exposed individuals. *Toxicol.* 188(2-3), 251– 259.

[60] Vaziri, N.D., Ding, Y., Ni, Z., Gonick, H.C., (1997). Altered nitric oxide metabolism and increased oxygen free radical activity in lead induced hypertension: effect of lazaroid therapy. *Kidney Intern.* 52(4), 1042–1046.

[61] Ding, Y., Vaziri, N.D., Gonick, H.C., (1998). Lead-induced hy-pertension. II. Response to sequential infusions of L-arginine, superoxide dismutase, and nitroprusside. *Environ. Res.* 76(2), 107–113.

[62] Bogden, J.D., Gertner, S.B., Kemp, F.W., McLeod, R., Bruening, K.S., Chung, H.R., (1991). Dietary lead and calcium: effects on blood pressure and renal neoplasia in Wistar rats. *J. Nutr.* 121(5), 718–728.

[63] Goldstein, G.W., Evidence that lead acts as a calcium substitute in second messenger metabolism. In: Proceedings of the 9th International Neurotoxicology Conference; October 1991, vol. 14 of Neurotoxicology. Little Rock, Ark, USA; 1993; pp. 97–101.

[64] Simons, T.J.B., Lead-calcium interactions in cellular lead toxicity. In: Proceedings of the 9th International Neurotoxicology Conference; October 1991, vol. 14 of Neurotoxicology. Little Rock, Ark, USA; 1996; pp.77–86.

[65] Duchen, M.R., (2000). Mitochondria and Ca^{2+} in cell physiology and pathophysiology. *Cell Calcium* 28(5-6), 339– 348.

[66] Chai, S., Webb, R.C., (1988). Effects of lead on vascular re-activity. *Environ. Health Persp.* 78, 85–89.

[67] DenHond, E., Nawrot, T., Staessen, J.A., (2002). The relationship between blood pressure and blood lead in NHANES III. National Health and Nutritional Survey. *J. Hum. Hypertens.* 16(8), 563–568.

[68] Bener, A., Obineche, E., Gillett, M., Pasha, M.A.H., Bishawi, B., (2001). Association between blood levels of lead, blood pressure and risk of diabetes and heart disease in workers. *Intern. Arch. Occupat. Environ. Health* 74(5), 375–378.

[69] Vupputuri, S., He, J., Muntner, P., Bazzano, L. A., Whelton, P.K., Batuman, V., (2003). Blood lead level is associated with elevated blood pressure in blacks. *Hypertens.* 41(3), 463–468.

[70] Rothenberg, S.J., Manalo, M., Jiang, Cuellar, R., Reyes, S., Sanchez, M., Diaz, M., Khan, F., Aguilar, A., Reynoso, B., Juaregui, M., Acosta, S., Johnson, C., (1999). Blood lead level and blood pressure during pregnancy in south central Los Angeles. *Arch. Environ. Health* 54(6), 382–389.

[71] Wang, X., Andrews, L., Riedel, S., Kaupp, M., (2007). Mercury Is a Transition Metal: The First Experimental Evidence for HgF4..*Angewandte Chemie Intern. Edit.* (Wiley-VCH) 46(44), 8371–5.

[72] US EPA (US Environmental Protection Agency), Mercury study report to Congress, vol. 7, Environmental Protection Agency, Washington, DC, USA; 1997.

[73] Cocoros, G., Cahn, P. H., Siler, W., (1973). Mercury concentrations in fish, plankton and water from three Western Atlantic estuaries. *J. Fish Biol.* 5(6), 641–647.

[74] Houston, M.C., The role of mercury and cadmium in cardiovascular disease, hypertension, and stroke. In: YV Li, JH Zhang, editor, Metal ion in stroke: Springer Series in Translational Stroke Research. New York: Springer; 2012; pp.767-782. ISBN 978-1-4419-9662-6

[75] Salonen, J.T., Seppänen, K., Lakka, T.A., Salonen, R., Kaplan, G.A., (2000). Mercury accumulation and accelerated progression of carotid atherosclerosis: a population-based prospective 4-year follow-up study in men in eastern Finland. *Atheroscler.* 148(2), 265–273.

[76] Huang, Y.L., Cheng, S.L., Lin, T.H., (1996). Lipid peroxidation in rats administrated with mercuric chloride. *Biol. Trace Elem. Res.* 52(2), 193–206, 1996.

[77] Lund, B.O., M.Miller, D., Woods, J.S., (1993). Studies on Hg(II)-induced H_2O_2 formation and oxidative stress in vivo and in vitro in rat kidneymitochondria. *Biochem. Pharmacol.* 45(10), 2017–2024.

[78] Guallar, E., Sanz-Gallardo, M.I., van't Veer, P., Bode, P., Aro, A., Gómez-Aracena, J., Kark, J.D., Riemersma, R.A., Martín-Moreno, J.M., Kok, F.J., (2002). Mercury, fish oils, and the risk of myocardial infarction. *N. Engl. J. Med.* 347(22), 1747N– 1754N.

[79] Salonen, J.T., Seppanen, K., Nyyssonen, K., Korpela, H., Kauhanen, J., Kantola, M., Tuomilehto, J., Esterbauer, H., Tatzber, F., Salonen, R., (1995). Intake of mercury from fish, lipid peroxidation, and the risk of myocardial infarction and coronary, cardiovascular, and any death in Eastern Finnishmen. *Circulation* 91(3), 645–655.

[80] Virtanen, J.K., Voutilainen, S., Rissanen, T.H., Mursu, J., Tuomainen, T.P., Korhonen, M.J., Valkonen, V.P., Seppänen, K., Laukkanen, J.A., Salonen, J.T., (2005). Mercury, fish oils, and risk of acute coronary events and cardiovascular disease, coronary heart disease, and all-cause mortality in men in Eastern Finland. *Arterioscler. Thromb. Vasc. Biol.* 25(1), 228–233.

[81] Rissanen, T., Voutilainen, S., Nyyssonen, K., Lakka, T.A., Salonen, J.T., (2000). Fish oil-derived fatty acids, docosahexaenoic acid and docosapentaenoic acid, and the risk of acute coronary events: the Kuopio Ischaemic Heart Disease Risk Factor Study. *Circulation* 102(22), 2677–2679.

[82] Yoshizawa, K., Rimm, E.B., Morris, J.S., Spate, V.L., Hsieh, C.C., Spiegelman, D., Stampfer, M.J., Willett, W.C., (2002). Mercury and the risk of coronary heart disease in men. *N. Engl. J. Med.* 347(22), 1755–1760.

[83] Hallgren, C.G., Hallmans, G., Jansson, J.H., Marklund, S.L., Huhtasaari, F., Schütz, A., Strömberg, U.,Vessby, B., Skerfving, S., (2001). Markers of high fish intake are associated with decreased risk of a first myocardial infarction. *Brit. J. Nutr.* 86(3), 397–404.

[84] Sørensen, N., Murata, K., Budtz-Jørgensen, E., Weihe, P., Grandjean, P., (1999). Prenatal methylmercury exposure as a cardiovascular risk factor at seven years of age. *Epidemiol.* 10(4), 370–375.

[85] Nakagawa, R., (1995). Concentration of mercury in hair of diseased people in Japan. *Chemosph.* 30(1), 135–140.

[86] Torres, A.D., Rai, A.N., Hardiek, M.L., (2000). Mercury Intoxication and Arterial Hypertension: Report of Two Patients and Review of the Literature. *Pediatr.* 105(3), E34. DOI: 10.1542/peds.105.3.e34

[87] Houston, M.C., (2011). Role of Mercury Toxicity in Hypertension, Cardiovascular Disease, and Stroke. *J. Clin. Hypertens.* 13(8), 621-7.

[88] Mozaffarian, D., Shi, P., Morris, J.S., Grandjean, P., Siscovick, D.S., Spiegelman, D., Willett, W.C., Rimm, E.B., Curhan, G.C., Forman, J.P., (2012). Mercury Exposure and Risk of Hypertension in US Men and Women in 2 Prospective Cohorts. *Hypertens.* 60, 645-652.

[89] Yonaha, M., Saito, M., Sagai, M., (1983). Stimulation of lipid peroxidation by methyl mercury in rats. *Life Sci.* 32(13), 1507–1514.

[90] InSug, O., Datar, S., Koch, C.J., Shapiro, I.M., Shenker, B.J., (1997). Mercuric compounds inhibit human monocyte function by inducing apoptosis: evidence for formation of reactive oxygen species, development of mitochondrial membrane permeability transition and loss of reductive reserve. *Toxicol.* 124(3), 211–224.

[91] Clarkson, T.W., (1972). The pharmacology of mercury com-pounds. *Ann. Rev. Pharmacol.* 12, 375–406.

[92] Lund, B.O., Miller, D.M., Woods, J.S., (1993). Studies on Hg(II)-induced H_2O_2 formation and oxidative stress in vivo and in vitro in rat kidneymitochondria. *Biochem. Pharmacol.* 45(10), 2017–2024.

[93] Gatti, R., Belletti, S., Uggeri, J., Vettori, M.V., Mutti, A., Scandroglio, R., Orlandini, G., (2004). Methylmercury cyto-toxicity in PC12 cells is mediated by primary glutathione depletion independent of excess reactive oxygen species generation. *Toxicol.* 204(2-3), 175–185.

[94] Kumar, S.V., Maitra, S., Bhattacharya, S., (2002). In vitro binding of inorganic mercury to the plasma membrane of rat platelet affects Na+-K+-ATPase activity and platelet aggregation. *BioMet.* 15(1), 51–57.

[95] Shumilla, J.A., Wetterhahn, K.E., Barchowsky, A., (1998). Inhibition of NF-κB binding to DNA by chromium, cadmium, mercury, zinc, and arsenite in vitro: evidence of a thiol mechanism. *Arch. Biochem. Biophys.* 349(2), 356–362.

[96] Kim, S.H., Johnson, V.J., Sharma, R.P., (2002). Mercury inhibits nitric oxide production but activates proinflammatory cytokine expression in murine macrophage: differential modulation of NF-kappaB and P38 MAPK signaling path-ways. *Nitr. Ox.* 7(1), 67–74.

[97] Willerson, J.T., Ridker, P.M., (2004). Inflammation as a cardiovascular risk factor. *Circulation* 109(no.21,suppl. 1), II2–II10.

[98] Holleman, A.F., Wiberg, E., Wiberg, N., Cadmium. *Lehrbuch der Anorganischen Chemie, 91–100* (in German). Walter de Gruyter; 1985; pp.1056–1057. ISBN 978-3-11-007511-3.

[99] Carballo, R., Castiñeras, A., Domínguez-Martin, A., García-Santos, I., Niclós-Guttiérrez, J., Chapter 7. Solid state structures of cadmium complexes with relevance to biological systems. In Astrid Sigel; Helmut Sigel; Roland K. O. Sigel. *Cadmium: From Toxicology to Essentiality*. Metal Ions in Life Sciences **11**. Springer; 2013; pp.145–189. doi:10.1007/978-94-007-5179-8_7

[100] EFSA., Cadmium dietary exposure in the European population. *EFSA J.* 10(1), 2551.

[101] FAO/WHO, Summary and conclusions of the seventy-third meeting of the Joint FAO/WHO Expert Committee on Food Additives, Geneva, 8–17 June 2010. Rome, Food and Agriculture Organization of the United Nations; Geneva, World Health Organization; 2010 (JECFA/73/SC;http://www.who.int/entity/foodsafety/publications/chem/summary73.pdf)].

[102] WHO, Cadmium. In: Guidelines for drinking-water quality, 3rd edition incorporating 1st and 2nd addenda. Vol. 1. Recommendations. Geneva, World Health Organization; 2008; pp.317– 319 (http://www.who.int/water_sanitation_health/dwq/GDW12rev1and2.pdf).

[103] Edwards, J.R., Prozialeck, W.C., (2009). Cadmium, diabetes and chronic kidney disease. *Toxicol. Appl. Pharmacol.* 238(3), 289–293.

[104] Gallagher, C.M., Meliker, J.R., (2010). Blood and urine cadmium, blood pressure, and hypertension: a systematic review and meta-analysis. *Environ. Health Persp.* 118(12), 1676–1684.

[105] Bernhard, D., Rossmann, A., Henderson, B., Kind, M., Seubert, A., Wick, G., (2006). Increased serum cadmium and strontium levels in young smokers: effects on arterial endothelial cell gene transcription. *Arterioscler. Thromb. Vasc. Biol.* 26(4), 833–838.

[106] Tellez-Plaza, M., Navas-Acien, A., Crainiceanu, C.M., Guallar, E., (2008). Cadmium exposure and hypertension in the 1999–2004 National Health and Nutrition Examination Survey (NHANES). *Environ. Health Persp.* 116(1), 51–56.

[107] Haswell-Elkins, M., Satarug, S., O'Rourke, P., Moore, M., Ng, J., McGrath, V., Walmby, M., (2008). Striking association between urinary cadmium level and albuminuria among Torres Strait Islander people with diabetes. *Environ. Res.* 106(3), 379–383.

[108] Schwartz, G.G., Il'Yasova, D., Ivanova, A., (2003). Urinary cadmium, impaired fasting glucose, and diabetes in the NHANES III. *Diabetes Care* 26(2), 468–470.

[109] Satarug, S., Nishijo, M., Lasker, J.M., Edwards, R.J., Moore, M.R., (2006). Kidney dysfunction and hypertension: role for cadmium, p450 and heme oxygenases? *Tohoku J. Exper. Med.* 208(3), 179–202.

[110] Sarkar, S., Yadav, P., Trivedi, R., Bansal, A.K., Bhatnagar, D., (1995). Cadmium-induced lipid peroxidation and the status of the antioxidant system in rat tissues. *J. Trace Elem. Med. Biol.* 9(3), 144–149.

[111] Menke, A., Muntner, P., Silbergeld, E.K., Platz, E.A., Guallar, E., (2009). Cadmium levels in urine andmortality among U.S. adults. *Environ. Health Persp.* 117(2), 190–196.

[112] Messner, B., Knoflach, M., Seubert, A., Ritsch, A., Pfaller, K., Henderson, B., Shen, Y.H., Zeller, I., Willeit, J., Laufer, G., Wick, G., Kiechl, S., Bernhard, D., (2009). Cadmium is a novel and independent risk factor for early atherosclerosis mechanisms and in vivo relevance. *Arterioscler. Thromb. Vasc. Biol.* 29(9), 1392–1398.

[113] Everett, C.J., Frithsen, I.L., (2008). Association of urinary cadmium and myocardial infarction. *Environ. Res.* 106(2), 284–286.

[114] Houtman, J.P., (1993). Prolonged low-level cadmium intake and atherosclerosis. *Sci. Total Environ.* 138(1–3), 31–36.

[115] Schutte, R., Nawrot, T., Richart, T., Thijs, L., Roels, H.A., Van Bortel, L.M., Struijker-Boudier, H., Staessen, J.A., (2008). Arterial structure and function and environmental exposure to cadmium. *Occup. Environ. Med.* 65(6), 412–419.

[116] Staessen, J.A., Kuznetsova, T., Roels, H.A., Emelianov, D., Fagard, R., (2000). Exposure to cadmium and conventional and ambulatory blood pressures in a prospective population study. Public Health and Environmental Exposure to Cadmium Study Group. *Am. J. Hypertens.* 13(2), 146–156.

[117] Nawrot, T., Den Hond, E., Thijs, L., Staessen, J.A., (2003). Isolated systolic hypertension and the risk of vascular disease. *Curr. Hypertens. Rep.* 5(5), 372–379.

[118] Whittemore, A.S., DiCiccio, Y., Provenzano, G., (1991). Urinary cadmium and blood pressure: results from the NHANES II Survey. *Environ. Health Persp.* 91, 133–140.

[119] Varoni, M.V., Palomba, D., Gianorso, S., Anania, V., (2003). Cadmium as an environmental factor of hypertension in animals: new perspectives on mechanisms. *Veter. Res. Commun.* 27(1), 807–810.

[120] Valko, M., Morris, H., Cronin, M.T., (2005). Metals, toxicity and oxidative stress. *Curr. Med. Chem.* 12(10), 1161–1208.

[121] Yiin, S.J., Chern, C.L., Sheu, J.Y., Tseng, W.C., Lin, T.H., (1999). Cadmium induced renal lipid peroxidation in rats and protection by selenium. *J. Toxicol. Environ. Health Part A* 57(6), 403–413.

[122] Steffensen, I.L., Mesna, O.J., Andruchow, E., Namork, E., Hylland, K., Andersen, R.A., (1994). Cytotoxicity and accumulation of Hg, Ag, Cd, Cu, Pb and Zn in human peripheral T and B lymphocytes and monocytes in vitro. *Gener. Pharmacol.* 25(8), 1621–1633.

[123] Wolf, M.B., Baynes, J.W., (2007). Cadmium and mercury cause an oxidative stress-induced endothelial dysfunction. *BioMet.* 20(1), 73–81.

[124] Abu-Hayyeh, S., Sian, M., Jones, K.G., Manuel, A., Powell, J.T., (2001). Cadmium accumulation in aortas of smokers. *Arterioscler. Thromb. Vasc. Biol.* 21(5), 863–867.

[125] Prozialeck, W.C., Edwards, J.R., Woods, J.M., (2006). The vascular endothelium as a target of cadmium toxicity. *Life Sci.* 79(16), 1493–1506.

[126] Prozialeck, W.C., Edwards, J.R., Nebert, D.W., Woods, J.M., Barchowsky, A., Atchison, W.D., (2008). The vascular system as a target of metal toxicity. *Toxicol. Sci.* 102(2), 207–218.

[127] Simovich, M.J., Conrad, M. E., Umbreit, J. N., Moore, E. G., Hainsworth, L.N., Smith, H.K., (2002). Cellular location of proteins related to iron absorption and transport. *Am. J. Hematol.* 69(3), 164–170.

[128] Kyselovic, J., Martinka, P., Batova, Z., Gazova, A., Godfraind, T., (2005). Calcium channel blocker inhibits western-type diet-evoked atherosclerosis development in apoE-deficient mice. *J. Pharmacol. Exper.Therap.* 315(1), 320–328.

Chapter 11

Conclusion and Future Research Need

It is concluded that there are several approved dietary risk factors for CVDs in our daily diets or foods. The dietary risk factors include toxicities caused by the over-intake of cholesterols, energy, SFAs, saccharides (especially fructose), irons, sodiums, alcohol, niacins, homocysteines, alkaloids (such as synephrines, caffeines, tyramines, dopamines, histamines, and cyanides), nucleic acids, trans-fatty acids, the metabolites of choline-containing compounds or L-carnitines and such environmental contaminants as leads, mercury or cadmiums; the deficiencies of folates, and vitamins D, B_6, or B_{12}; the toxicity or deficiency of magnesiums; and the consumption of sweetened soft drinks. An underweight, or even normal weight, might not decrease the occurrence of CVDs because the deficiency of some nutrients, and alkaloids in above mentioned chapters that are able to control the weight, could also damage the cardiovascular system.

It seems that the association of all these risk factors in the blood with CVDs, has been well established though some minor controversial opinions on some risk factors exist. And also, their levels in the blood are likely associated with their dietary intakes. Therefore, it should be worth carrying out further studies to investigate the correlation between these risk factors in foods or diets and their levels in the blood as well as the occurrence of CVDs.

Most importantly, it seems that the data of dietary safety of these risk factors is based on the test on a single factor. What would the cardiovascular system undergo if a person is used to have his daily foods that contain all cardiovascular risk factors for a long time? Is any unknown CVD risk component present in our daily diets? It is worth undertaking extensive research to answer these questions. Especially, the cooperative effects of the CVD risk factors on the cardiovascular system need to be studied well, even though the concentration of each in our daily foods might be safe for consumption. For example, the test on a prepared diet or food containing all the risk factors for CVDs discussed in this book should have a prospective outcome and contribute a lot to the prevention of CVDs in the future.

In addition, it has been reported that there are digoxin-like factors in some kinds of foods or diets. And also, the association of the digoxin-like factors with CVDs has been indicated. For example, digoxin-like factors were found to cause bradycardia and hypotension [1], though they have been employed as medicines to enhance the heart performance. The digoxin (1.2 ng/mL in the blood and higher) may harm patients with a heart failure [2,3]. Its levels >2 ng/mL in the blood are commonly toxic, but it may have toxicity at lower levels [4]. Furthermore, the digoxin especially harms patients who have significant sinus or atrioventricular block [4]. More cautiously, a target range of 0.5-1.0 ng/dL in blood has been recommended [5].

The digoxin-like factor is defined as the chemical compound that has an effect on the cardiovascular system similar to that of the digoxin. The structure of this class of compounds has not yet be understood.

The action of the digoxin is primarily associated with the inhibited Na^+/K^+ ATPase, mostly in the myocardium. The inhibited Na^+/K^+ ATPase results in an elevated concentration of sodiums inside the cells, leading to the sodium-calcium exchanger acting reversely so that the normal action of transporting 3 extracellular Na^+ into the cell and 1 intracellular Ca^{2+} out of the cell was shifted to an reversed action that elevates the levels of the intracellular Ca^{2+} ready for the contractile proteins.

The increased intracellular calciums lengthen the phase 0 and phase 4 of the cardiac action potential so that the heart rate is reduced [6]. The elevated intrcellular calciums can also result in the elevation of the Ca^{2+} storage in the sarcoplasmic reticulum, leading to an elevated calcium release during every action potential so that the heart contractility is increased without elevating the expenditure of energy in the heart. Thirdly, the inhibited sodium pump might have a positive effect on the sensitivity of baroreceptors in patients with a heart failure[7]. Furthermore, the digoxin may have parasympathetic effects, especially on the atrioventricular node [8].

The action of the degoxin therefore causes the reduced heart rate accompanied by an elevated blood pressure, leading to a net elevation of volume of each stroke volume and an elevated perfusion of tissues. This can improve the efficiency of the myocardium, accompanied by the optimization of hemodynamics and an improved curve of ventricular function in patients with a heart failure. Furthermore, the digoxin was found to elevate the vagal activity which slows the depolarization of pacemaker cells in the atrioventricular node and therefore the heart rate [9]. Because of this property, the digoxin is often employed in treating different kinds of arrhythmias. However, it seems that it is difficult to find reports on discussing whether these actions of the degoxin are good for a healthy heart or not.

Moreover, the degoxin has other electrical effects. For example, the action potential can be initially elevated by the degoxin and then the conductance of K^+ is reduced because of the elevated level of the intracellular Ca^{2+}. This could cause the reduction of refractory period of the ventricles and atria as well as the elevation of the atrioventricular and sinoatrial nodes, which can result in a smaller negative resting potential in membranes and thus elevated irritability.

The information about the content of the digoxin-like factors in foods seems to be nearly absent from the literature. However, the intake of a herbal tea caused toxicity because of the increased level of plasma digoxins that were mainly contributed by the components of cayenne pepper fruits and hops flowers [1]. The author reported that 4.85, 2.51, 1.84, 0.656, 0.579, and 0.555 μg digoxin equivalents/200 mL cup of the tea were contributed by cayenne peppers, hops, skullcaps, wood betonys, valerians, and black cohosh, respectively. The cayenne pepper is eaten as a daily vegetable by many people in the world, especially by most Chinese. The hops flower is an essential ingredient for making beer. Are those compounds in these foods or their products, having the effects on the vascular system similar to the degoxin, are really degoxins? Are they present in other foods? It should be worth carrying out further studies to answer these questions.

References

[1] Scheinost, M.E., (2001). Digoxin toxicity in a 26-year-old woman taking a herbal dietary supplement. *J. Am. Osteop. Assoc.* 101(8), 444-6.

[2] Adamson, P.B., Suarez, J., Ellis, E., Kanaly, T., Vanoli, E., (2004). Ephedrine increases ventricular arrhythmias in conscious dogs after myocardial infarction. *J. Am. Coll. Cardiol.* 44(8), 1675-8.

[3] Chan, K.E., Lazarus, J.M., Hakim, R.M., (2010). Digoxin associates with mortality in ESRD. *J. Am. Soc. Nephrol.* 21, 1550–9.

[4] Dec, G.W., (2003). Digoxin remains useful in the management of chronic heart failure. *Med. Clin. North. Am.* 87(2), 317-37.

[5] Hunt, S.A., Abraham, W.T., Chin, M.H., Feldman, A.M., Francis, G.S., Ganiats, T.G., Jessup, M., Konstam, M.A., Mancini, D.M., Michl, K., Oates, J.A., Rahko, P.S., Silver, M.A., Stevenson, L.W., Yancy, C.W., (2009). 2009 focused update incorporated into the ACC/AHA 2005 Guidelines for the diagnosis and management of heart failure in adults. *Circulation* 119, e391–e479.

[6] Tripathi, K.D., *Essentials of Medical Pharmacology* (6th ed.). New Delhi: Jaypee Publications; 2008; pp.498. ISBN 81-8448-085-7.

[7] Wang, W., Chen, J,S., Zucker, I.H., (1990). Carotid sinus baroreceptor sensitivity in experimental heart failure. *Circulation* 81(6), 1959–66.

[8] Gheorghiade, M., Adams, K.F., Colucci, W.S., (2004). Digoxin in the management of cardiovascular disorders. *Circulation* 109(24), 2959–64.

[9] Goodman, D.J., Rossen, R.M., Cannom, D.S., Rider, A.K., Harrison, D.C., (1975). Effect of digoxin on atioventricular conduction. Studies in patients with and without cardiac autonomic innervation. *Circulation* 51(2), 251–256.

Author's Contact Information

Professor Dr. Wenbiao Wu
College of Food Science, Southwest University,
216 Tian Sheng Qiao, Beibei,
Chongqing PRC
Email: wbwu62@yahoo.com

Index

#

A

B

C

D

E

F

G

H

I

J

K

L

M

N

O

P

Q

R

T

U

V

W

X

Y

Z